SURGEON, HEAL THYSELF

Optimising Surgical
Performance by Managing Stress

SURGEON, HEAL THYSELF

Optimising Surgical Performance by Managing Stress

Uttam Shiralkar, MS, FRCS, MRCPsych

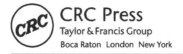

CRC Press
Taylor & Francis Group
Boca Raton London New York

CRC Press is an imprint of the
Taylor & Francis Group, an **informa** business

CRC Press
Taylor & Francis Group
6000 Broken Sound Parkway NW, Suite 300
Boca Raton, FL 33487-2742

© 2017 by Taylor & Francis Group, LLC
CRC Press is an imprint of Taylor & Francis Group, an Informa business

No claim to original U.S. Government works

Printed on acid-free paper in Great Britain by Ashford Colour Press Ltd
Version Date: 20170110

International Standard Book Number-13: 978-1-4987-2403-6 (Paperback)

Library of Congress Cataloging-in-Publication Data

Names: Shiralkar, Uttam, author.
Title: Surgeon heal thyself : optimising surgical performance by reducing stress / Uttam Shiralkar.
Description: Boca Raton : CRC Press, [2016] | Includes bibliographical references and index.
Identifiers: LCCN 2016051738 (print) | LCCN 2016052667 (ebook) | ISBN 9781498724036 (paperback : alk. paper) | ISBN 9781498724043 (eBook PDF)
Subjects: | MESH: Stress, Psychological | Surgeons--psychology | Surgical Procedures, Operative--psychology | Clinical Competence
Classification: LCC RD27.5 (print) | LCC RD27.5 (ebook) | NLM WM 172.4 | DDC 617/.0232--dc23
LC record available at https://lccn.loc.gov/2016051738

Visit the Taylor & Francis Web site at
http://www.taylorandfrancis.com

and the CRC Press Web site at
http://www.crcpress.com

Contents

Acknowledgements

I would like to thank Jonathan Earnshaw, Paul Wilson, Mike Hallissey, Snehal Patel and Anupama Shrotri for providing valuable feedback after reading the manuscript. I would like to offer special thanks to my friend and spinal surgeon from the USA, Ravi Vedantum, for providing feedback and contributing with his anecdotal information. I would also like to thank Duncan Learmonth for preparing the cognitive simulation script.

I would like to thank all the editorial staff at CRC Press as, without their help, this book would not have been possible.

We gratefully acknowledge the permissions granted to reuse material from the following.

- Groopman J. *How Doctors Think*. New York: Houghton Mifflin Company; 2007. Reproduced with permission from Dr Jerome Groopman MD.
- Abernathy C.M., Hamm R.M. *Surgical Scripts*. Philadelphia: Hanley & Belfus; 1994. Reproduced with permission from Dr Hamm.

About the author

Uttam Shiralkar qualified and worked as a surgeon for 15 years in the UK, India and USA, before entering the field of psychological medicine. A developing interest in psycho-oncology and the medical problems he faced after a car accident were some of the reasons that contributed to this move.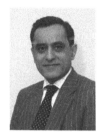

While pursuing a career in psychological medicine, it became clear to him just how much of an impact a surgeon's psychology could have on clinical outcomes. He felt the need for surgeons to be made aware of this issue in a bid to address some of the shortcomings of the current system of surgical practice. To share this knowledge, he authored his first book titled *Smart Surgeons, Sharp Decisions*.

A good-quality surgery is said to have two key elements: safe judgement and good technical skills. The first book was about the first part: the judgement. It was well received by surgeons in various part of the world and the British Medical Association (BMA) awarded it a 'highly commended book' prize. The *Journal of the American Medical Association* (JAMA) and the *ANZ Journal of Surgery*, among other journals, also had complimentary words to say.

This was more than enough encouragement for Dr Shiralkar to set about writing on the second key element for successful surgery: the technical skills. In this book, titled *Cognitive Simulation*, he wrote on the importance of cognitive factors and how surgeons can use cognition to improve operative skills.

Currently, in addition to fulfilling his commitment as a consultant in the NHS, Uttam is actively involved in coaching surgeons at various levels of their careers on a range of issues, providing mentorship, conducting research, speaking at meetings and conducting workshops.

CHAPTER 1

Preface

An on-call surgeon was asked to see a patient in the accident and emergency unit. The patient was an obese woman in her thirties who was involved in a car accident. She was unconscious, her skin was pale and blood was seeping from her nose. The surgeon found her tachycardiac, hypotensive and breathing rapidly. He also noted that, even with an oxygen mask at full flow, her oxygen saturation was not adequate. To make sure that the patient's airway was not blocked, he placed the oxygen mask over the mouth and pressed the bellows. The oxygen level rose to 98%. He realised that the patient needed endotracheal intubation and requested the on-call anaesthetist, Dr Jones, to carry out an immediate intubation. Dr Jones took the laryngoscope and pushed the blade through the patient's mouth. Unable to see into the larynx due to collected blood, Dr Jones put in the suction cannula and brought up a cupful of clotted blood. When she tried to insert the endotracheal tube, the oxygen saturation started falling, going down to 70%. Attempts to push the tube further proved futile and the patient became cyanosed. When the saturation fell to 60%, Dr Jones pulled the tube out and put back the mask. Shortly, the oximeter reading went up to 97%. After a while, when she tried to insert the tube again, the oxygen saturation dropped as before, and the mask was put back once more. However, this time the saturation did not go up and the patient started becoming cyanosed in spite of being under the mask with full oxygen flow.

Realising the critical situation, the surgeon called for a tracheostomy set, a brighter light and an experienced assistant from another operating room. Amid the buzz of hectic activity in this stressful situation, he tried to remain calm. He reassured himself that the tracheostomy was going to be a straightforward procedure, as he just needed to make an incision through the cricothyroid membrane. With that thought, he placed his fingers to locate the edge of the patient's thyroid cartilage, but due to the thick fat around the neck, he was unable to feel through it. That made him feel uncertain and hesitant, exactly what a surgeon is not supposed to experience in these situations! He was conscious that time was running out and four minutes without oxygen would leave the patient with brain damage.

Grasping the scalpel, the surgeon made a quick incision. As the assistant held the retractors, he started dissecting with scissors but struck a vein. Immediately blood filled the wound and it became difficult to see the operative field. Suction was necessary but the apparatus was clogged from the previous use. An additional overhead light was brought in but it still was not bright enough. He had to mop up the blood with gauze and, feeling around with his fingertips, palpated the ridge of the thyroid cartilage and the gap of the cricothyroid membrane below. He then forced the blade down on the thyroid cartilage and cut through with small, sharp strokes, though blood and poor light obscured the wound. When the blade scraped against bony cartilage, he worked the tip into a gap he thought was the cricothyroid membrane. As the tissue gave way, he made an opening. As the surgeon tried to insert the tracheostomy tube, he felt some blockage and had to twist, turn and jam it in. The ventilation tubing was attached to the tracheostomy tube but when the bellows was pressed, the air burbled out of the wound! The tracheostomy tube was not in the trachea! The patient had been without an airway for about three minutes. Meanwhile the patient's saturation had dropped below detection point. Her heart rate started dropping and within a few seconds the pulse disappeared! The surgeon put his hands on the patient's chest and began giving chest compressions. Just then the anaesthetist managed to insert a paediatric-size endotracheal tube into the vocal cords and establish the airway. In a few seconds the patient responded, her pulse returned, the saturation started improving. All the people in the room exhaled, as if they, too, had been denied their breaths.

I have retold above the stressful operative situation that Dr Atul Gawande eloquently depicted in his book *Complications*.[1] You may have experienced similar incidences or have heard comparable stories. Over the last 15 years, I have gathered a great deal of understanding regarding how surgeons manage stress in the operating room. This understanding is based on interacting with surgeons across specialties, seniority and nationalities. I have also made specific observations about master surgeons and noticed what these top surgeons do differently from the rest. I found, apart from knowledge and technical skills, that what helps these master surgeons most is the way they handle stress more effectively in critical situations and deliver better clinical outcomes.

I did not stop with anecdotal opinions based on what I saw but went through evidence-based studies to support or refute the views. Studies have been carried out to assess surgeons' performance in stressful situations. Researchers have systematically collected observations about surgeons' behaviour and performance from a range of sources, including physiological monitoring, self-reported questionnaires and other objective investigations. This allows us to know how a surgeon deals with stress by analysing a range of objective parameters rather than just trusting our perception.

It's not just surgeons who experience performance-related stress. I have scanned through research on other aspects of performing under stress from similar demanding professions such as aviation, the military and sports. All the information gathered has one common conclusion: beyond a certain level, stress is detrimental to a satisfactory performance outcome. It weakens performance and sets the stage for failure. Under stress, it is not only surgeons, but also the likes of pilots and air traffic controllers, law enforcement officers, and others in highly stressful circumstances, who make errors in judgement. Internationally reputed athletes miss their well-practised shots under stress. Business leaders, when under extreme stress, make poor decisions. Stress is not just any other adversary for a performer; it is a landmine in a career path, waiting for you to put your foot on it. In this book I will elaborate on some of the findings that I have gathered in the last 15 years.

There are many attributes that make a surgeon successful. Attributes like knowledge, judgement and decision making are the most important. Whether you are choosing an appropriate procedure for a patient or making sense of investigations you carried out, stress negatively impacts your thinking and will affect decisions. In addition to affecting thinking, stress downgrades psychomotor skills. Any performer, be it a musician or an athlete, will tell you that psychomotor performance is compromised under excessive stress. We can observe this in our everyday skill of driving. You may have observed a car driver trying to make a U-turn on a busy, narrow street. The driver will feel under stress from an impatient truck driver behind her who cannot go around until she makes the turn. She is likely to hit the curb or stall the car, taking longer than usual if the truck driver starts expressing his impatience by blowing the horn. This further delays the irked truck driver and causes embarrassment for the car driver.

In extremely stressful moments, many surgeons perform below their capability. Counterintuitively, researchers have revealed that when people are desperate to do their best, they fail to do so. Statistics have proven these points by showing that professional sportspeople rarely perform better than their average in pressure moments and some, even the elite, do worse. You may not realise the damaging effect of stress on your performance as many other factors often mask it. You may think you made an incorrect decision because you did not have the necessary information, but the reality may be that due to the stress, you were unable to access the information even though it was available. When you have tried various ways to improve your performance, without much success, you should consider the possibility that inadequate stress management could be holding you back.

Today, we feel increased stress in our professional lives. Surgeons across specialties and regions live in a high-pressure atmosphere, where on each working day they may feel that as though their lives are 'on the line'. More than before, practising surgeons feel that they have to work harder, perform better and have better outcomes. Every decision they make or procedure they perform may seem to have a bearing on their career. A negative outcome can create problems in an atmosphere where anything can damage the surgeon's professional reputation that has been earned with years of hard work and great outcomes.

There are various reasons for increased stress in the surgical profession: information overload, administrative pressures, technological advances, complexities of the surgical procedures and political atmosphere, among others. Some surgeons have reached a point where they say, 'In the morning when I start driving from my home to my operating list, I wonder if I will be able to do the cases without any major problems.' This can be seen as 'performance anxiety', fear about whether you are able to perform satisfactorily. Nowadays we see the risk of performance anxiety extending to other areas of our lives. The ongoing sensation that you will have to perform at your best and the underlying reservations as to whether you can perform as expected lead to stressed exchanges and strained relationships in personal lives. As a consequence of stress, the surgeon's spouse often experiences the 'short-fused' surgeon unleashing stress on family members. At times, these problems become so unmanageable that interpersonal conflict becomes a regular event. Suddenly, the middle-aged surgeon starts feeling as though he or she is under siege on every front. In view of the fact that surgeons work longer hours and that the surgical field is becoming more competitive, stress has become a plague in the current professional environment.

An observation that surprises me is that a significant number of surgeons with whom I have interacted take a casual approach to managing stress in their professional lives. Very few of them appear to think about how to handle stressful situations better until it is too late. Very few have strategies that are in line with the current scientific understanding of stress management. Like many surgeons over the decades, they simply model what they have observed from their trainers or mentors and hope it works. Do not get me wrong, these strategies can work, but many times they don't.

Traditionally, surgeons suppress feelings of stress as part of their training. They have also been indoctrinated to believe that expression of feelings of stress is a sign of weakness and unbecoming to a good surgeon. Some surgical residency programmes are similar to military training in which constant stress is considered an essential part of the training itself. As a result, most surgeons withhold and bottle up their feelings and emotions of stress. In addition, several teachers and mentors in male-dominated surgical specialties like orthopaedic surgery have traditionally frowned upon trainees who display stress-related emotional feelings. The result is that a majority of surgeons are left feeling helpless as to how to vent their stress-related feelings and emotions.

My purpose in writing this book is twofold. First, to provide a user-friendly and easy-to-read book on stress management specifically aimed at surgeons – practical strategies that individual surgeon can use. The second purpose is to inoculate surgeons against the detrimental effects of stress, so that they can perform to their maximum potential in critical moments such as during a complex procedure, an intraoperative complication or a high-stakes case.

It is expected that by managing stress during surgical performance, the patient outcome will improve. However, one needs to be clear on one thing: The success of stress management should not be judged solely by the outcome. With the management of stress, the best you can do is your best, which for a particular case may not be good enough. Managing stress allows you to perform closer to your potential and this increases the chances of a successful outcome. Managing stress puts you in a position to experience a successful outcome because it allows experience, knowledge and skills to do the talking without holding you back.

This concept is supported by research done in various disciplines, including aviation, business, and the military, as well as medicine and surgery, in particular. It shows that training people to cope with stress in their professional lives is an unused strategy for unleashing their capabilities. Further, this strategy helps them perform at their true proficiency rather than having it compromised due to stress. This book provides the tools for developing the coping skills that allow a surgeon to do his/her best even in the most stressful situations.

The more conversant you are with the effect of stress on performance, the more skilful you are likely to become at coping with it. This book provides readers with some powerful stress-management strategies that can be used when they are involved in a critical situation or are anticipating one in the near future. Some of the solutions can be applied immediately. These solutions are described in Chapters 8 and 11, so if you are currently in the midst of a stressful situation and if you feel ill equipped to handle it, look at this section now for a 'quick fix'. Chapters 9 and 10 offer long-term strategies to help build confidence, optimism and tenacity. With these techniques, you can immunise yourself against distress so that your capability is not reduced by it. We have found this strategy to be lacking in many surgeons, even the experienced ones. Even if you feel that you are good at handling stress, the information in this book will help you to share the knowledge with other surgeons who may benefit from your experience and will appreciate your help.

Almost all surgeons undergo stress in their work and yet they have to perform in the face of it. With the strategies described in this book, I have observed that, over time, they realise that while mustering knowledge and technical skills provides them with basic requirements, their real ticket to success comes from being able to cope well under stress. The information in this book has given surgeons specific solutions, as well as helped them prepare long-term coping strategies to better deal with stressful incidents. It is hoped that it will also help you, not just in critical moments but also in any situation that matters in your clinical life.

You will be able to apply the cutting-edge information from what is provided by cognitive science. In stressful situations, you will have less distorted thinking, less indecisiveness and more creative ideas. I believe that when you enter an operating room to perform a very complex procedure, you will see that as more of a challenge than as a crisis, and you will come out a feeling that you performed to the best of your capabilities.

REFERENCE

1 Gawande A. *Complications: a surgeon's notes on an imperfect science.* New York: Henry Holt & Company; 2002.

CHAPTER 2

Why should we pay heed to stressed surgeons?

No aspect of life is more stressful than work-related stress. This is not surprising, considering the importance of a career in our lives. Work provides us with purpose and is linked to our personal identity. A significant number of us do not work simply to earn a living but for personal satisfaction. The number of people reporting high levels of work-related stress has more than doubled in the last few years. The United Nations has recognised occupational stress as 'The 20th Century Disease' and the World Health Organization has described job-related stress as a worldwide epidemic.[1]

Although stress is an issue for people in every field, it is more prevalent among medical professionals due to factors integral to care-giving work. The problems of stress among health professionals have been highlighted in recent years. Surgery has been further singled out as putting people at higher risk. Despite its significant impact, not enough progress has been made in preventing core issues related to work stress in surgery. Although it is perceived to be one of the most stressful of all medical specialties, proportionally, there is little in surgical literature that has specifically explored this issue.

A stratified cross-sectional survey of doctors was carried out in Canada to compare the levels of distress among the major medical specialties. The responses revealed that emergency physicians and surgeons reported the highest levels of distress, while administrative physicians and community health specialists reported the lowest. Thus the survey confirmed the perception that surgery is one of the most stressful disciplines.[2]

Surgery is physically demanding and intellectually challenging. A surgeon's evening may be filled with the residual stress from the day's happenings; a procedure may have been unexpectedly difficult, a patient in an intensive care unit may have developed a complication, the morbidity and mortality meeting may have been embarrassing, and interaction with a resentful patient may have generated a sense of helplessness.

Stress is so pervasive in surgery that it is not a matter of whether surgeons will experience stress, but of when and how. Moreover, there are many different ways in which surgeons experience stress and individual variations in experiencing the stress are more important; i.e. 'how' is more important than 'when'. These variations contribute significantly to the degree of distress experienced by an individual. Being highly driven professionals, surgeons have attributes that make them more vulnerable to stress. Individuals who are compulsive and have high standards of performance are attracted to surgical specialties. Common terms used to describe surgeons are inflexible, controlling and perfectionist, features of Type A personality. This personality characterises driven and high-achieving individuals. They are impatient and assertive. Those who display more of these Type A personality attributes are likely to experience more difficulty coping with stress. Attributes like dedication, although desirable as a professional, increase susceptibility to stress.[3] Surgeons are reputed to be fiercely competitive, with assertive tendencies such that the working atmosphere can be described as 'cut-throat'. Some surgeons are very difficult to get along with and are too critical of others. People manage to put up with them, not because of their position, but because some of them know that these surgeons are even harder on themselves. As they say, 'sparse on compliments and ruthless in self-criticism'.

There was a very busy and well-known surgeon in the USA, Dr CK, who displayed compassion, kindness and a caring attitude to his co-workers and patients, whether seeing patients in the office or in the hospital. However, his demeanour in the operating room was a whole different story. It was not uncommon for him to yell, shout, demand and be rude to his co-workers. In the operating room, as the day went on, he would become increasingly agitated and unpredictable in his

behaviour towards co-workers. His co-workers all knew not to make
any small talk when he was doing surgery. He would sometimes come
out of the operating room after finishing a case, and grab hold of
the hand-washing sink and shake it violently while simultaneously
grunting and making growling noises. This habit of shaking the
hand-washing sink continued until one day he overheard a co-worker
jovially discussing the possibility of loosening some of the screws on
the sink so that the next time Dr CK tried to shake the sink it would
come loose from the wall.

Traditionally surgeons have displayed attributes as independent doers, always ready to act. They prefer not to ask for help, say 'thank you', or to have much trust in anything outside of their own abilities. They work hard, expect perfection and do not accept excuses. To the trainees, some surgeon mentors are decent human beings while others are tyrants. Personalities aside, surgeons use their hard-earned physical skills to get results in the operating theatre. They rely on themselves for success or failure. They are the captains of their ships. Surgery is a specialty of instant gratification, for patient and surgeon alike.

According to Thomas Krizek, a well-known American plastic surgeon, surgery is not just combination of medicine and technical skills. Surgery has its own set of psychological demands that define the nature of the surgeon. Surgery is thrilling, but it is not for everyone. Surgeons experience exhilaration while performing technically demanding interventions. While doing so, they take risks. The excitement of performance gets balanced against the frustration of failure. Some surgical specialties derive satisfaction from life-and-death challenges, others by improving a bodily function. Nonetheless all of surgery involves action; action involves risk and risk entails stress. Despite the fact that surgeons are chosen from hundreds of intelligent medical graduates, there are still those who do not posses the required psychological attributes.[4]

There is another contributing factor in a surgeon's stress. From the day we begin cadaveric dissection in anatomy, we start a distinctive association with the human body. This unusual association separates surgeons from all other professionals who function at the border of human relationships and intimacy. Surgery is special. Surgeons and their patients cannot avoid intense personal contact. The people surgeons encounter are at their most vulnerable. Patients trust the surgeon with paramount responsibility. Dealing responsibly with the sick, the injured, the terminally ill and those in pain exacts an emotional toll on surgeons, although they may not be aware of it. As Thomas Krizek says, 'Some become hardened by the experience; empathy gets depleted. Dealings with patients become scripted rather than felt.'[4] Some become emotionally empty while others become stressed.

Surgeons' detachment from patients can be seen as a necessary defence. It may be that if surgeons were to empathise with their patients who are in fear, in pain or dying, it may aggravate their own stress and their efficiency as surgeons may be compromised. Therein lies the rub for all who walk the line between necessary detachment and appropriate intimacy with patients. A surgeon needs to be able to step away from the bright operating lights, away from the invisible patient wrapped under the drapes – and later sit at the patient's bedside for an empathetic exchange that the patient expects. Juggling between these two contrasting roles can be stressful.[5]

We observe high variability in individual responses to the same stresses and individual characteristics, such as coping style, are more significant than the nature of the work stress itself. Although there are some stresses inherent to the nature of a surgeon's work, the effect varies depending on the individual. Thus, the stress experienced by a given individual in a situation is highly dependent on individual tendencies. The key to effective stress management lies in self-awareness and recognition of the triggers. Identifying the sources of stress and modifying the stressors is a strategy in minimising stress. For a surgeon stress is inevitable, but it should not be uncontrollable.[3]

Although the impact of chronic stress has been acknowledged, the psychological entity of acute stress has not been acknowledged proportionally. This is especially significant for surgeons, since integration of complex cognitive processes with manual dexterity is vital for performing safe procedures. Dealing with critically ill patients and life-threatening incidents causes considerable stress on the surgeon. This is set against a background of a working atmosphere troubled by distractions and poor teamwork.

Approximately 243 million surgical procedures are performed each year worldwide.[6] Although the risk of complication is often low, adverse events do occur. Almost half of these adverse events are considered to be preventable. To reduce the occurrence of preventable complications, nowadays emphasis has been placed on improving the dynamics within the operating room – the human factors. Additionally, the use of checklists and pre- and post-operation debriefing has been appraised.

Although progress is being made to improve the quality of surgical performance, unfortunately little attention has been paid to the relationship between a surgeon's stress and performance under pressure. Although some surgeons are aware that there is significant variation among individual surgeons' performance during stressful situations, this has remained a personal view and the factors underlying varied ability are not evaluated in a systematic way. If differences do exist, these most likely will have an impact on patients. For these reasons, a better understanding of the factors behind these differences is necessary. Indeed, other disciplines in which performance under pressure is required have extensively studied factors that have led to improved outcomes.

Aviation and military sectors have recognised that stress has significant effect on performance. Soldiers are being offered specific training to deal with the stress. Like the military and aviation, surgery is a safety-critical field. However, unlike those fields, the effects of stress among surgeons are rarely recognised. Both pilots and surgeons are expected not to commit any error while performing their tasks. In aviation, perceptions of stress and error are included as topics of formal training. The work culture in aviation has evolved in such manner that it addresses any error in an effective and appropriate manner. In contrast, surgical culture has evolved to cover up errors. Surgeons as a group find it hard to accept vulnerability to error. They have a tendency to play down the effects of stress and fatigue. This is not an anecdotal view but a conclusion from the studies that have compared pilots and surgeons. When pilots' attitudes on stress and errors were compared with those held by surgeons, differences in attitudes regarding stress were obvious: Surgeons are in the habit of denying the effects of fatigue and stress on performance but pilots are not. A study found 70% of surgeons refuted the effect of fatigue on performance, compared with only 26% of pilots.[7] The denial of stress and its effects on performance may help individuals adjust during surgical training, but a healthy recognition of stressor effects reduces the likelihood of error later in a surgeon's career. Exhausted pilots who recognise their own boundaries cope with their stress and fatigue by requesting crewmembers to keep an eye on them or transferring the assignment to somebody else. Many disasters, such as flying accidents, military defeats and incidents on the space station are related to the failure of a performer to execute routine actions under stress.[8] Research has shown that individuals can be trained to recognise stress as an error inducer and the self-acknowledgement continues to improve with coaching.[9]

In the old system of training, surgeons used to take whatever fatigue, abuse and work came their way. They used to learn how to keep moving forward despite mental and physical stress. Mistakes did occur; yet the situation carried on and the system did work for some surgeons. It forced them to dig deep and find out what they were made of, especially in a critical situation when blood was squirting from the operative site and no one was around to help. In those days, despite the unconscionable hours and exhaustion, the on-call resident used to get excited when a trauma patient arrived in the middle of the night, knowing they would get a chance to operate independently.

Some experienced surgeons have reservations about the surgeons coming out of training today. The specific concerns relate to lack of experience handling intraoperative stress. According to them, most of the best (and worst) work was done in the 100th or 120th hour of the week. The best work was gratifying; the worst work was at least character building. The jury is still out regarding the experience of surgeons coming out of training today; as a result of recent reforms, are they less experienced than the generation before? There is no doubt that surgical trainees have a better quality of life today. But the concern remains whether they are as competent to handle the intraoperative stress as their trainers are.

In the old days, those who ran the surgical departments were giants in their field and they ran the department with a strong fist. That was how *they* had been taught. One can say that they passed their own past sufferings to the next generation. They were supreme in their kingdom and were not keen to give up their pearls of wisdom without a mental price. These were not user-friendly teaching schemes but inhumane tests of stress endurance. In addition to the brutal workload, often the trainees had to face verbal abuse from those who were meant to shape them. Everything was the resident's fault, regardless of the fact. If your boss was operating and cut into the wrong artery, it was your fault for not alerting the surgeon. If a patient under your boss had a setback on the ward, again, it was your fault for not looking after the patient. You just had to adapt to every situation without any complaint. Complications after surgery or a death were deemed personal failures.

During the training period resident surgeons used to meet interesting mentors who guided their surgical hand. They came in all shapes and sizes, and with a variety of egos and skills. Time and energy were scarce commodities and emotions had to be buried. There was never any time to dwell on anything but the task directly in front of you. Displaying emotions was a sign of weakness. Across the systems, surgical training is more humane today than it was in years past. The actual, intentional physical and emotional abuse that prevailed for years is long gone; it simply won't be tolerated in this day and age. However, the other side of the change is that we need to provide alternative mechanisms to develop resilience among surgeons. The first step in developing resilience is to establish whether surgery is stressful for surgeons or not. The next chapter will reveal if that is the case.

SUMMARY

Although stress is an issue for people in every field, it is more prevalent among doctors and surgeons have been further singled out as being at an even higher risk. Stress is so pervasive in surgery that it is not a matter of whether surgeons will experience stress, but of when and how much. Being highly driven professionals, surgeons have attributes that make them more vulnerable to stress. We observe high variability in individual responses to the same stresses and individual characteristics such as coping style have a greater effect than the nature of the stress itself. Stress experienced by a surgeon while performing a procedure is a vital aspect of surgical performance and the management of intraoperative stress, which affects clinical outcome directly, is a key component of a surgeon's competence. Disciplines like aviation and the military, which are considered to be high-reliability and safety-critical industries, have long recognised that even the expert performers are susceptible to rapid deterioration in performance under stress. They did not just acknowledge this factor but have started suitable training programmes to moderate its effects. Surgery has yet to catch up with these developments. The first step in the right direction would be to acknowledge the role of stress in surgery.

REFERENCES

1 *Protecting workers. Health Series No. 6: raising awareness of stress at work in developing countries.* World Health Organization; 2007.
2 Lepnurm R., Lockhart W.S., Keegan D. A measure of daily distress in practicing medicine. *Can J Psychiatry.* 2009; 54(3): 170–80.
3 Laporta L.D. Occupational stress in oral and maxillofacial surgeons:

tendencies, traits, and triggers. *Oral Maxillofac Surg Clin North Am.* 2010; 22(4): 495–502.

4 Krizek T.J. The impaired surgical resident. *Surg Clin North Am.* 2004; 84: 1587–1604.

5 Page D. Are surgeons capable of introspection? *Surg Clin North Am.* 2011; 91: 293–304.

6 Weiser T.G., Regenbogen S.E., Thompson K.D., Haynes A.B., et al. An estimation of global volume of surgery, a modelling strategy based on available data. *Lancet.* 2008; 372: 139–44.

7 Sexton J.B., Thomas E.J., Helmreich R.L. Error, stress, and teamwork in medicine and aviation: cross sectional surveys. *BMJ.* 2000; 320(7237): 745–9.

8 Sandal GM. The effects of personality and interpersonal relations on crew performance during space simulation studies. *Int J Life Support Biosphere Sci.* 1999; 5: 226–37.

9 Merritt A.C., Helmreich R.L. CRM: I hate it, what is it? (Error, stress, and culture). In: *Proceedings of the Orient Airlines Association Air Safety Seminar, 23–25 April 1997, Jakarta, Indonesia.* Manila: Orient Airlines Association; 1997. pp. 123–34.

CHAPTER 3

Is performing surgery really stressful?

The operating room is not just a sterile milieu but also a sacred space. The surgeon enters into a privileged relationship with the patient, one of the most intimate that anyone can think of. Although the operating milieu relies heavily on technology, those around the operating table should not ignore the impact on the patient. The patient is as helpless as any human being can be: To begin with, stripped naked; then we place the person in a setting with its own rules that everyone except the patient knows about. Additionally, we take away any control that the person has. To top it off, we anesthetise, and thus make him totally surrender. For the surgeon, the total submission of the patient is expected to heighten the sense of responsibility. Each motion of dissection should be a small return to the patient for the surrender of autonomy. Essentially a contract, albeit unwritten, needs to be followed: Every patient would be offered the best planning, the best technique, the best operation and – above all – the best state of mind of the surgeon at the time of performing.[1]

If a group of surgeons are asked a simple question, 'Do you feel stressed while operating?', you will get range of answers, from 'Not at all' to 'Yes, too much'. There are many reasons behind this variability of responses. First, the term *stress* is applied too liberally and non-specifically. It may reflect different experiences to different individuals. Second, it may be difficult to specify what stress is. This leads to a third reason: difficulty in identifying it. Then comes the fourth reason: There is no clear-cut demarcation between when the experience of stress is good and when it is not. In addition, the level of complexity of the surgery itself, experience in doing the procedure, expectations of patient and family, as well as the familiarity of the surgeon with equipment, surgical staff and operating room, may all contribute to the presence or absence of the sense of stress for the surgeon. For all these reasons, surgeons generally have difficulty in acknowledging stress and its potential impact on their performance. Moreover, stress is seen as a weakness. Since it is seen as a failing, nobody would like to admit it. Additionally, many believe that stress is an inevitable part of their work; therefore, they have to tolerate it.[2] They also like to think they can deal with stress in any situation.

Before we think of other reasons for the lack of acknowledgement about stress among surgeons, let us try to find out what stress means for surgeons and how it can be identified better. Time-based understanding can first reduce the complexity of the concept of stress. A simple division between chronic stress and acute stress will make it little easier to understand. Thus for the sake of the present discussion, let us divide the 'stress' into 'acute' and 'chronic'.

Where else do surgeons experience acute stress other than in the operating theatre? The operating room is a very demanding environment. It is the place where surgeons spend approximately one-third of their working time.[3] To get a clearer idea, let us see if there is any evidence of surgeons experiencing stress in the operation room. Since the aim here is to highlight how serious the issue of stress is among surgeons, the focus is going to be on the evidence-based information. It will thus underline that stress is not just a 'touchy-feely' matter; rather, it is a significant issue of which every surgeon needs to be aware.

Surgeons perform physically and mentally stressful procedures, some more frequently than others. However, we do not know how demanding such operations are with respect to psychophysical stress. Surgeons use considerable muscle force while performing operations. They use instruments that are not always light in weight – an additional factor for increased stress on the cardiovascular system. For these reasons it would be useful to know how a surgeon's physiological parameters change while performing a surgery.

Bergovee and Orlic explored whether surgeons' cardiovascular responses, expressed as metabolic equivalents (METs), increase during an operating procedure and if any particular parts of the procedures are more challenging than others.[4] They also tried to determine whether surgeons' cardiovascular responses changed according to age or experience. Orthopaedic surgeons with operative experience varying from less than 100 procedures to more than 1000 procedures took part in the study. The procedure to be observed was the first operation on the list and expected to be of average difficulty. A blood pressure monitor and a Holter ECG recorder monitored the surgeons while they were performing procedures. According to the surgeon's activity and the instruments used, key points were considered as either physically less demanding or more demanding. When a surgeon was using forceps, scissors and needle holder it was considered to be 'less demanding', while the use of mallet, oscillating saw or bone-cutting forceps was considered to be 'more demanding'. METs were calculated to reflect the energy requirements and psychophysical stress for the activities. The results obtained during the procedure were compared with the standard METs during everyday activities.

Results showed that when compared with everyday activities, the average energy requirements of performing the operation were equivalent to moderate-intensity physical activity (Figure 3.1).

The amount of energy surgeons spent was less than 2.5 METs in the 30-minute period before and after the procedure, which is similar to activities like walking at a slow pace, making a bed, playing a musical instrument or sweeping a floor. The energy consumed for the less-demanding parts of the procedure was between 2.5 and 3 METs, which is the amount of energy used in slow dancing, fishing, or walking

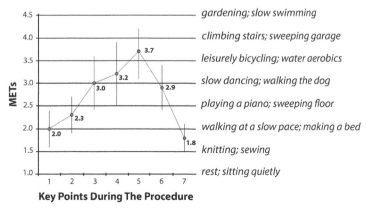

Figure 3.1 Energy requirements of operating compared with everyday activities[4]

the dog. Between 3 and 4 METs were needed during physically more demanding parts, equivalent to water aerobics, golf, walking at an average pace, leisurely bicycling, climbing stairs, or playing table tennis. The energy requirements of the demanding part of the operation required approximately 40% of a surgeon's cardiovascular maximum.

While looking at these findings we need to keep in mind that this energy expenditure was for the first operation of the day that was of average difficulty. Surely, surgeons perform more challenging operations and also more than one operation in a day. In cases where complications happen or when the surgeon has already performed some operations, the energy spent is likely to be higher. Other factors may increase surgeons' psychophysical stress while operating, like additional work breathing, resulting from airway resistance and heat caused by masks, occlusive garments, and lights.

This study revealed one unexpected observation: There was no difference in cardiovascular response according to a surgeon's prior operative experience or seniority. We would expect that intraoperative stress decreases with experience. These findings challenged that assumption. This unexpected finding could be explained by considering the difference in physical strength between senior and junior surgeons. Senior surgeons may be less psychologically stressed than junior surgeons, but they also have less muscular strength and therefore may have to expend more physical effort.

Seven surgeons in the study developed cardiac arrhythmias during the operations, which was another unexpected finding. Psychological stress is a known risk factor for development of cardiac arrhythmia. This may be a reason why, when looking at cardiovascular mortality among doctors, surgeons are at higher risk of cardiac mortality. In the context of cardiovascular parameters, performing procedures that equal moderate-intensity physical activity may be equated with recreational bicycling. The psychophysical status of the surgeon while performing physically demanding procedures could be compared with the psychophysical condition of athletes in a competitive challenge. The rise in cardiovascular parameters in both cases is due to physical activity as well as to psychological stress.

How does operative stress compare with the other professional activities and how does the stress of the operation change when activities such as teaching are involved? To answer these questions a study was carried out which compared the surgeon's blood pressure (BP) while operating in three different situations: trainee assisting the trainer; trainer assisting the trainee; and trainee operating independently. The changes in BP and heart rate of surgeons during the operation day were compared with their BP and heart rate changes during a clinic day.[5] As we all know, blood pressure and pulse rate are routinely measured on patients undergoing surgical procedure. However, we have not paid attention to what happens to the surgeon's BP while operating on the patient!

Half of the surgeons were experienced and the remaining half consisted of residents. The surgeons were monitored during a total of 21 elective surgeries. Each trainer and trainee pair wore the ambulatory BP monitor for 3 days. There were two operating days and one control day. The control day was a day spent in the outpatient clinic.

The study found that mean arterial pressure (MAP) and heart rate increased showing peaks and troughs according to the technically challenging parts of the procedure. When the trainer was the operating surgeon, her MAP started rising preoperatively and remained high until the critical phase of the procedure passed, settling thereafter. When the trainer was assisting the trainee, MAP readings for the trainers were consistently high. Thus the trainer was apprehensive throughout the procedure when the trainee was performing. At the same time the trainees' BP was consistently higher while performing than when they were assisting. The highest MAP recordings were when trainees operated independently; understandably, that is when they are most stressed. Also, compared with the average BP recording on clinic days, the average BP on an operating day was higher. While it cannot be concluded from this single study that training a surgeon induces hypertension in the trainer, it seems that trainees may be inducing episodic hypertension! However, this is likely to settle as the experience of the surgeon increases.

One may think that the stress is observed while the surgeon is performing life-saving or major procedures only. The study carried out by Yamamoto and colleagues challenges that view. They showed that intraoperative stress is seen during a routine cataract surgery as well.[6] In the study, stress was assessed by measuring heart rates and urine adrenaline levels. Surgeons were divided into three categories according to their surgical experience:

1. Inexperienced – fewer than 100 cases
2. Intermediate – 100 to 500 cases
3. Experienced – more than 500 cases.

The inexperienced surgeons had the highest heart rates at the beginning of surgery but the rates decreased towards the end of the procedure. All values of stress markers in inexperienced surgeons were higher than those of the other two groups throughout the procedure. In surgeons with intermediate experience, heart rates were not as high as in the inexperienced personnel; however, they were higher than normal throughout the surgery. The heart rate of intermediate surgeons did rise significantly when the procedure was to be broadcast live on closed-circuit television. Measurements of experienced surgeons were only marginally higher. Thus the variations in heart rates and urine adrenaline levels showed characteristic patterns based on the experience of the surgeons. Unlike the previously mentioned study in which the experienced surgeons had similar cardiovascular changes as the inexperienced, the findings of this study supported the conventional view that operative stress reduces with experience.

You may be aware that some physiological changes seen as a result of stress are similar to the changes seen due to fatigue. Looking at that, one may say that the observations could be due to fatigue rather than to stress. One may go a step further and say that the stress could be secondary to fatigue itself. However, fatigue as a factor affecting intraoperative stress can be ruled out when you notice that the heart rates of the surgeons decreased towards the end of surgery. If the increase in the heart rate had been due to fatigue, the heart rate may have stayed stable or increased near the end of the procedure. Also, the heart rates of very experienced surgeons started closer to normal and remained almost flat throughout the surgery, which would not have happened if fatigue had caused these changes. Furthermore, the heart rates and urine adrenaline levels of a highly experienced surgeon did not differ between the first and the seventh consecutive surgeries on the same day.

It is noteworthy that the postoperative urine adrenaline level of the surgeon who performed surgery during a closed-circuit television demonstration was four times that of the normal value, similar to the values of a sample obtained from a novice pilot flying a jet. Simultaneous television demonstration of surgery is gaining in popularity. However, these observations suggest that the surgeon's experience should be considered before the system is used. Highly experienced surgeons were minimally affected by the television demonstration. Another interesting observation was that inexperienced surgeons became stressed as soon as they entered the operating room. Senior surgeons may be able to acknowledge this issue and modulate their behaviour to minimise the high stress at the beginning of surgery.

If teaching and performing a cataract surgery induce stress as above, one can only imagine the stress of performing and teaching cardiac surgery. The manner in which attending consultant surgeons educate trainees, in critical specialties like cardiothoracic surgery, remains an issue for discussion. Teaching trainee cardiac surgeons without affecting the surgical results is challenging. Supervising and assisting trainees is in some cases mentally more demanding than performing. A group of researchers studied the intraoperative heart rate variability (HRV) of the attending consultant surgeon as a measure of psychological stress.[7] They wanted to know if there were any differences in the HRV when an attending consultant surgeon performed coronary artery bypass grafting surgery and when he assisted. We know that cardiac surgeons are always under pressure to yield satisfactory results for both the patients and referring cardiologists.

Heart rate variability is the physiological phenomenon of variation in the time interval between heartbeats. It is measured by the variation in the beat-to-beat interval. According to some experts, measuring HRV is currently one of the best methods of assessing stress and is more sensitive than measuring heart rate alone. HRV measures the balance between sympathetic and parasympathetic systems. The parasympathetic activity is the main contributor of high-frequency (HF) power in HRV while increase in the low-frequency (LF) power is a measure of sympathetic activity. The low frequency/high frequency ratio mirrors the sympathetic/parasympathetic balance. When sympathetic activity increases, the LF power increases; conversely, when vagal activity increases, HF power increases. Therefore, it is useful to calculate the LF:HF ratio, in which a lower ratio indicates better adaptability. The normal value of the LF:HF ratio is 1.5–2.0.

This study was the first to evaluate the intraoperative cardiac changes of a cardiac surgeon while performing bypass surgery. Fifty cases of coronary artery bypass grafting were observed. An attending consultant surgeon performed 30 procedures (Group A) and supervised the remaining 20 cases performed by resident surgeons (Group B). The entire procedure was divided into six steps to evaluate the most demanding parts of the procedure and to compare the two groups.

Two specific observations were noted. First, the LF:HF ratio of the attending consulting surgeon was highest during the earlier part of the procedures and it stabilised and decreased towards the end. Second, the LF:HF ratio was highest in the heart arrested and coronary anastomosis phase when he supervised a resident trainee surgeon as an assistant. These observations suggest two things: First, in the hands of an attending consultant surgeon, once the operation begins the stress tends to decrease and the surgeon then becomes relaxed. Second, an attending consultant surgeon automatically pays more attention to the specific steps of the procedure such as arresting the heart, coronary arteriotomy and sewing coronary grafts when she supervises a resident trainee surgeon because she knows those phases are the most important steps. Thus it showed that there is a clear difference in the experience of stress when a surgeon performs a procedure than when she supervises.

A Swedish study found that surgeons are at an increased risk of death from ischaemic heart disease than the general population. The major difference between the studied populations was in regard to work characteristics. Surgeons work at a faster pace, their schedules are hectic, they are unable to relax after work, and their work is also physically demanding. The increase in sympathetic activity during surgery may have deleterious effects, ranging from worsening of ischaemia to lethal arrhythmias or sudden death.[8]

The psychological stress results in cardiovascular and metabolic effects in the form of an 'alarm reaction' which prepares a subsequent physical reaction. Metabolically or energetically 'non-consumed' stress is known to cause health hazards. The effect of unconsumed psychological stress is the opposite of physical stress, as physical exercise is a metabolically 'consumed' stress. Sympathetic arousal is the precipitator of myocardial ischaemia during mental stress. Parasympathetic activity predominance is in some way protective, not only with respect to cardiovascular morbidity, but also with respect to general survival. One well-defined implication of these studies is that 'stressful' experiences, if sustained by surgeons with marginal cardiac reserve, could precipitate cardiac pathology if this degree of sympathetic hyperactivity is prolonged. This observation urges us to consider such cardiac diseases as occupation-related illnesses, for which surgeons should make allowances.[9]

SURGEONS DO NOT GET TO CHOOSE – PEACEFUL REST OR REST IN PEACE

Heart rate variability is useful not just for diagnosis; it has a prognostic value as well. In the general population, low HRV has been associated with increased risk of cardiac events. We have seen that surgeons experience stress during an operation but we do not know if similar changes are seen during on-call night shifts. Amirian and colleagues evaluated the HRV of surgeons during night shifts.[10] No other study has investigated the HRV during an entire 17-hour night shift by surgeons. The results showed a change in autonomic nervous system activity, with sympathetic dominance during the on-call period. The HF values were high on the pre-call night compared with those on the on-call night, indicating a higher vagal influence. The surgeons had a significantly higher pulse rate during the 17 hours they worked on a night shift, which supported the findings of sympathetic dominance. While on call, the increase in LF:HF ratio demonstrated a sympathetic dominance. The overall findings demonstrated surgeons' stress response regardless of training levels. The study also showed that surgeons had decreased HRV during on-call hours, as the vagal activity was significantly reduced. These findings are noteworthy as the HRV monitoring was carried out continuously during both pre-call and on-call duration, providing solid insight on the sympathetic-parasympathetic balance of the entire recording period.

Stress experienced by on-call surgeons is a known reality that has been supported by the above study. However, after this period of studied observation, there is another real-life situation that surgeons face: operating after the night on call. Yamaguchi assessed surgeons' stress from night duty and surgery.[11] Another aspect of this study that differs from earlier studies is the inclusion of subjective stress assessment in addition to the objective measure. The validated questionnaires 'Stress Arousal Checklist' (SACL) and 'NASA Task Load index' (TLX) were used for subjective assessment of stress. The objective parameter was the amount of biopyrrin in the urine. Biopyrrin is one of the bilirubin oxidative metabolites in urine and its urinary concentrations are increased after stress.

The subjective stress score after the operation showed that stress increased in proportion to the increase in duration of the surgery and to the amount of surgical blood loss. Similar changes were seen in biopyrrin levels. The increase in the level was proportional to the duration of surgery; the longer the duration, the higher the levels. Biopyrrin levels also increased after an operation when the blood loss was more than 200 mL. The levels were significantly elevated the morning after night duty and decreased after the following day shifts.

With measures in place to reduce the stress of residents, attending surgeons have to bear more responsibilities when on call. Some senior surgeons stop accepting night duties while others ask for additional remuneration to offset the stress. Thus, commercial systems can offer some financial compensation to the stress. However, money cannot prevent the physical toll. It is said that lack of sleep for 24 hours has a similar effect to having a blood alcohol concentration of 0.10%. At this level, driving is considered to be unsafe. Fewer than 6 hours of sleep during night call duty is associated with increased incidence of complications in procedures carried out by surgeons. There is a view that the sleep-deprived surgeon is ethically obligated to rest before performing a complex procedure. Although research has found the biomarkers of sleep deprivation, a test for pathological sleep deprivation, like the alcohol Breathalyser, is not yet available. Until such a test is available the onus is on surgeons to make judicious decisions about their fitness to operate. Successive night shifts affect alertness, metabolism and the general sense of well-being. We do not know the long-term effects of sustained night duty on a surgeon's longevity. Just as frequent acute stress can end up becoming chronic stress, similar effects are likely to occur in the case of sleep deprivation.

The unique feature of this study was the combination of subjective and objective assessments of stress. Although it showed that both parameters were affected by stress, a more robust methodology would be convincing. This is why a recent study by Rieger and colleagues is helpful. They examined the cardiovascular effects of stressed as well as non-stressed surgeons by measuring heart rate and heart rate variability.[12]

The surgeons were assigned to stressed or non-stressed groups according to their subjective stress scores. It was expected that the individual stress experience would be reflected in the cardiac tests. In this respect, the researchers analysed whether there were any differences in HR and HRV between intraoperatively stressed and non-stressed surgeons. Ambulatory monitoring of the surgeon was carried out for 24 hours under normal working conditions. The stress questionnaire (State Trait Anxiety Inventory – STAI) was used immediately before and after the operative procedure. Intraoperative stress was indicated if the postoperative score was higher than the preoperative. Based on that, surgeons were divided into stressed and non-stressed groups.

Nearly half of the group experienced stress during the procedure. Intraoperative HR differed significantly between stressed and non-stressed surgeons. The night-time HRV was different as well. Relative HR changes between surgery and night-time showed significant differences between stressed and non-stressed surgeons. In stressed surgeons, HR increased by 63.6%, whereas in the non-stressed group it was raised by only 34.6%.

Reduced or stationary HRV indicates reduced autonomic adaptability during recovery. Non-stressed surgeons showed greater adaptability; however, HRV of stressed surgeons remained unchanged, reflecting poor recovery after stressful events. The prognostic value of HRV after myocardial infarction in reduced HRV has proven its association with mortality risk in seemingly healthy individuals. It was observed that stressors were related to higher HR and lower HRV during awakening and that the effects of stressors were extended into the night recovery.

One of the advantages of this study was that measurements were performed during the routine work schedule without any external interference. Nevertheless, real-world findings are subject to influence by unrelated factors. A surgeon's physical fitness is one such factor. However, among the participants the fitness was at a high level in both groups of surgeons. Thus tachycardia seen in stressed surgeons was not due to poor fitness. Likewise, both groups operated under similar working conditions. So tachycardia within the stressed group is unlikely to be the result of metabolic variances, but rather due to the combination of muscular and mental strain.

One of the difficulties in assessing the impact of stress is the variability of methods that have been used to assess the stress. Because stress is a complex issue, different groups or individuals have chosen different measures according to their preferences. To address this problem, researchers at Imperial College, London developed a tool, the Imperial Stress Assessment Tool (ISAT), that captures stress from three perspectives.[13] A unique aspect of this tool is that the objective assessment covers both systems affected by stress: cardiovascular and neuroendocrine. The ISAT consists of simultaneous administration of three stress measures:

1. Salivary cortisol (objective components) – salivary cortisol is a non-intrusive marker of stress and an accurate indicator of serum cortisol

2. Continuous heart rate monitoring (objective components)

3. Self-reported stress levels (subjective component).

Although each of these measures has been independently proven as an indicator of stress, it is the first time they have been used together as a combined assessment tool with surgeons. It is thought that HR is more sensitive, but cortisol more specific in detecting stress. The two components of ISAT are thus complementary.

During this study, 54 operations by 11 surgeons were monitored. Surgeons were from general surgery, cardiothoracic and orthopaedic departments. A wide range of procedures was included. Twenty-three out of 54 procedures were perceived as stressful by the surgeons and increased HR and cortisol levels were found in 80% of these stressful procedures. That nearly half of the procedures were stressful highlights the fact that stress during surgery is a real issue and more common than surgeons acknowledge.

So far we have seen various studies, employing various methods, that endeavoured to confirm whether surgeons experience stress while operating. We saw questionnaires being used, biological markers being assessed and cardiac monitoring being done – all to examine the experience of stress from various angles. However, if we keep a narrow focus on objectivity and protocols, we miss a simple but very effective way to understand the complex issue of stress – asking surgeons for their point of view. That was the approach in a qualitative study to explore surgeons' perceptions of surgical stress.[14] The researchers chose an interview-based approach to explore surgeons' perceptions. Surgeons in London, both trainees as well as practising surgeons, offered their views on this issue.

Surgeons' attitudes to highlight the positively challenging features of their work was obvious during the early part of the interview. Some of them, mostly very experienced surgeons, claimed that stress was not a problem for them. Further questions like 'How do you manage to stay calm during emergencies or surgical complication?' revealed that most surgeons experience stress, but those who handle it successfully do not think it is a problem. However, most of the surgeons accepted that stress was a very important factor in their work. When asked to give an account of what it feels like when stressed, they portrayed their personal experiences. All those experiences could be grouped into four specific domains, as follows.

1. **Physical reactions:** 'When stressed you get the feeling of adrenaline rush' a surgeon said. He described heart pounding, sweating and physical tension while operating under stress. When specifically asked about the effects of stress on operative skill, surgeons reported feeling shaky, clumsy and less skilful. As a result, they made small mistakes such as placing the stitches inappropriately.

2. **Emotional reactions:** Emotions experienced by the surgeons were varied, such as anxiety, anger, frustration and irritation. Resident surgeons experienced difficulty ascertaining their own competence and ambiguity concerning when to call for help in critical situations.

3. **Cognitive reactions:** Many surgeons found it difficult to think clearly under stress. They had difficulty analysing problems in a logical manner and found it challenging to make decisions about how to proceed further in the operation. Some surgeons experienced urgency to think, high pressure and a tendency to rush to a decision. Surgeons start suspecting their own previous decisions or experience dilemmas between two strategies. Distractive thoughts start troubling them, such as worries about justification of the surgery, their reputation, or medicolegal problems.

4. **Behavioural reactions:** Although the frustrated surgeon throwing instruments in the middle of an operation is rare in recent years, these surgeons acknowledged that they become short tempered while facing a stressful situation. Actions which were otherwise straight-forward appeared problematic. Ideally, during stressful situations the communication within the team should be facilitative. In reality, surgeons experience worsening of communication patterns in such situations.

All the evidence-based information provided above is expected to make you aware of the seriousness of operative stress. However, being aware is insufficient. Many people are aware that smoking kills, but they just don't acknowledge that it may or will hit them one day. So one must acknowledge that it, may happen to them, too. Similarly, beyond becoming aware, a surgeon needs to acknowledge the impact of stress on his performance.

SUMMARY

Although surgeons experience various stressors while performing a procedure, they are more likely to deny the effects of stress than other professionals experiencing similar stress in their work. Because of this attitude, researchers have stayed away from investigating this issue in more depth and in a robust manner. As a result of insufficient research, organisational and educational change in policies has not taken place. At the same time, it must be acknowledged that the currently available research has shown without doubt that stress is a significant factor in surgical practice that should not be ignored by the surgical fraternity. No single best measure exists to evaluate stress directly. Therefore, the only way to estimate the level of stress is by measuring its effects, either on surgeon's perceptions or on her physiological changes. Various questionnaires that are easy to administer have been designed and validated to evaluate the level of subjective stress. Cardiac and biochemical investigations have provided complementary evidence of the stress surgeons experience while operating.

REFERENCES

1 Schwaitzberg S.D., Godinez C., Kavic S.M., Sutton E., et al. Training and working in high-stakes environments: lessons learned and problems shared by aviators and surgeons. Perspective of a surgeon educator/trainer. *Surg Innov.* 2009; 16(2): 187–95.

2 Arora S., Sevdalis N., Nestel D., Tierney T., et al. Managing intraoperative stress: what do surgeons want from a crisis training program? *Am J Surgery.* 2009; 197: 537–43.

3 Rieger A., Stoll R., Kreuzfeld S., Behrens K., Weippert M. Heart rate and heart rate variability as indirect markers of surgeons' intraoperative stress. *Int Arch Occup Environ Health.* 2014; 87(2): 165–74.

4 Bergovee M., Orlic D. Orthopaedic surgeons' cardiovascular response during total hip arthroplasty. *Clin Orthop Relat Res.* 2008; 466: 411–16.

5 Gupta H.O., Gupta S., Carter R.L., Mohammed A., et al. Does orthopedic surgical training induce hypertension? A pilot study. *Clin Orthop Relat Res.* 2012; 470: 3253–60.

6 Yamamoto K., Hara T., Kikuchi K., Hara T., Fujiwara T. Intra-operative stress experienced by surgeons and assistants. *Ophthalmic Surg Lasers.* 1999; 30: 27–30.

7 Song M-H., Tokuda Y., Nakayama T., Sato M., Hattori K. Intraoperative

heart rate variability of a cardiac surgeon himself in coronary artery bypass grafting surgery. *Interact Cardiovasc Thorac Surg.* 2009; 8: 639–41.

8 Arnetz B.B., Andreasson S., Strandberg M., Eneroth P., Kallner A. Comparison between surgeons and general practitioners with respect to cardiovascular and psychological risk factors among physicians. *Scand J Work Environ Health.* 1988; 14(2): 118–24.

9 Demirtas Y., Tulmac M., Yavuzer R., Yalcin R., et al. Plastic surgeon's life: marvelous for mind, exhausting for body. *Plast Reconstr Surg.* 2004; 114(4): 923–30.

10 Amirian I., Andersen I.T., Rosenberg J., Gogenur I. Decreased heart rate variability in surgeons during night shifts. *Can J Surg.* 2014: 57(5): 300–4.

11 Yamaguchi K., Kanemitsu S. Surgeons' stress from surgery and night duty: a multi-institutional study. *Arch Surg.* 2011; 146(3): 271–8.

12 Rieger A., Stoll R., Kreuzfeld S., Behrens K., Weippert M. Heart rate and heart rate variability as indirect markers of surgeons' intraoperative stress. *Int Arch Occup Environ Health.* 2014; 87: 165–74.

13 Arora S., Tierney T., Sevdalis N., Aggarwal R., et al. The Imperial Stress Assessment Tool (ISAT): a feasible, reliable and valid approach to measuring stress in the operating room. *World J Surg.* 2010, 34: 1756–63.

14 Wetzel C.M., Kneebone R.L., Wolosynowych M., Nestel D., et al. The effects of stress on surgical performance. *Am J Surg.* 2006; 191: 5–10.

.

CHAPTER 4

Effects of stress on surgical performance

Surgeons use skills in a high-stakes environment where death can be the worst outcome for the patient. In aviation, pilots use their skill to fly where death can be the worst outcome for the passengers as well as for the pilot. In both cases, perfection is pursued in a high-stakes environment with a flawed tool: the human mind. There are some more parallels between a surgeon and a pilot. The aviator will fly a heavy, complex machine costing millions, navigate it through three-dimensional space, manoeuvring it through hazardous environments, and return it intact to the ground. The surgeon will enter the patient's body, navigate through complex anatomy, perform risky procedures and bring the patient safely out of the operating room. Though the specific tasks and skills are different, the challenges that pilots and surgeons face as they master their craft are remarkably similar.[1] Just as there are similarities, there are differences. Perhaps the most remarkable are the differences that exist in their attitude to the effect of stress on their performance. Pilots seem to have more insight into the effects of stress on their performance and are proactive in making changes in their work accordingly. Most surgeons, on the other hand, do not wholeheartedly acknowledge the impact of stress on their performance. Although there may be awareness among some surgeons that a high level of stress is associated with poor dexterity, any link between the two has not been studied and proven strongly, thus not appreciated by many, which again reflects lack of regard for this issue among surgeons. Here we will go through the evidence about the effect of stress on surgical performance.

Let us look at the first-ever study that was carried out to see if stress does impair surgical performance.[2] The worsened performance was observed in the longer time required for the manoeuvres, poorer economy of motion, and increased number of errors.

Surgeons who had assisted in a minimum of five laparoscopic cholecystectomies but had not performed this procedure independently took part in the study. The participants were asked to perform three simple tasks on a simulator.

- The first task involved 'Transfer Place', which consists of grasping a virtual sphere with one hand and transferring it to the other.
- The second task, 'Manipulate Diathermy', involved boxes that appear around the sphere to be cauterised by touching them with the diathermy in one hand while holding the sphere steady in the other hand.
- The skills from both the first and second tasks were combined to form the third task, 'Withdraw and Insert', where the sphere is held steady with one hand and is touched with the instrument held in the opposite hand, which is then reinserted as a diathermy and touches the boxes around the sphere again.

Assessment of the entire task was tracked and recorded by the simulator for time taken to complete the task, economy of movements and number of errors for each hand.

Stress was measured using the Imperial Stress Assessment Tool (ISAT) in a triangulated approach. For subjective assessment, the State Trait Anxiety Inventory (STAI), which measures emotional, cognitive and physical stress, was administered. STAI consists of six items on a four-point scale, which participants use to self-report how stressed they felt before, during and after the laparoscopic task (minimum score = 6, maximum = 24).

An objective assessment was carried out using salivary cortisol immediately before and after participants completed the laparoscopic task. Recording the heart rate was part of the objective assessment. The surgeons wore a heart rate monitor during the entire period of performing the task.

The subjective and objective measurements of stress were in agreement with each other. Thus objective tests did indeed capture mental stress and the changes in the parameter were not due to the physical activity. Furthermore, heart rate and cortisol changes occurred in a complementary manner: an increase in the heart rate was related to an increase in the level of cortisol. All stress tests revealed that the participating surgeons were most stressed while performing the procedure. With regards to the performance, the greater the stress, the more likely it was that the surgeon would make an error, the longer he took to complete the task and the higher number of unnecessary movements were made. Not only did the objective parameters correlate with the worsened performance, but the subjective experience of stress also correlated with the number of errors and economy of motion. This shows that for a surgeon, especially for an inexperienced one, performing a simple but novel task causes stress to the degree that the qualities of even simple actions are detrimentally affected.

It is understandable that an inexperienced surgeon may experience stress while learning a new skill. However, one may wonder what effects a stressor has on experienced surgeons. To find that out, we need to look at the study done by Schuetz, Gockel and colleagues.[3] This was the first study to examine surgeon-specific stress reactions using a sympathicograph in stressful situations. The researchers wanted to find out if stress responses are associated with changes in surgical skills and errors of the surgeons who have experience in laparoscopic surgery. The activity of the sympathetic nervous system was monitored through skin resistance. The changes in the skin resistance were recorded with the help of a sympathicograph.

Electrodes of the sympathicograph were placed on the neck of the participating surgeons. The number of laparoscopic operations previously performed by the participating surgeons was divided as follows:

1. Fewer than 10 procedures
2. Between 10 and 49 procedures
3. Between 50 and 99 procedures
4. More than 100 procedures.

In the course of the study, the surgeons were exposed to four different stresses (S1–S4), in defined intervals:

S1 – at 3 minutes, after the start of virtual cholecystectomy; a mathematical task is given to solve.

S2 – at 6 minutes, critical information is given by the anaesthesiologist; substantial loss of blood occurs during the operation; there is time pressure to terminate the procedure.

S3 – at 9 minutes, sound volume of the pulse oximeter of the patient increases; at the same time, tachycardia accelerates.

S4 – at 12 minutes, a representative of the regional chamber of physicians arrives to find out details of the course of the procedure.

All stress reactions were categorised into three types according to the graphic presentation on sympathogram. The three surgeon-specific stress reactions (SSR) were as follows:

SSR-1: This type of reaction was observed in 22% of surgeons. There was a significant degree of stress reactions without any recovery even after the stressors stopped.

SSR-2: This type was observed in 39% of surgeons and showed full recovery after the stress reactions.

SSR-3: The remaining 39% of surgeons did not show any significant stress reactions.

Thus it could be said that approximately two-thirds of surgeons experienced stress while performing, some of them recovered after the procedure, some didn't. After looking at the above findings one may think that the effect of stress on surgical performance is intuitively detrimental, but that effect has not been quantified in a robust manner. This may have happened because, until lately, it has been tough to assess surgical dexterity. The availability of simulators and motion-analysis systems has helped make an objective assessment of surgical skills possible. Due to the availability of objective means for assessment of surgical skills we can now assess the effect of adverse conditions on surgical performance. The following study used sophisticated technology to study the effect on surgical skill more accurately.[4] As part of an experiment to see the effects of various types of stress on performance, surgeons with different levels of experience were asked to perform a laparoscopic transfer task.

Surgeons were asked to move cylindrical pieces of sponge from one disc to another on a laparoscopic simulator. The task was performed under five different stress-inducing conditions:

Q: quiet conditions, no stressor

N: background operating theatre noise at 80 to 85 decibels (dB)

M: simultaneous performance of a simple mental arithmetic task

T: performance as quickly as possible

A: all three stressors applied in combination.

Surgical performance was assessed using a motion-analysis system. The dexterity was measured by motion-tracking sensors attached to the dorsum of both hands.

When the trackers are placed on the hands move in an electromagnetic field of the motion-analysis system, it gives information on the number of movements and the path length traversed by each hand. It provides information regarding accuracy, total path length, and path length per movement. Path length is the total path traversed by the hand during the performance of the task. Path length per movement is the average path length traversed by the hands with each movement.

The results showed that a significantly higher number of errors occurred under all four stress-inducing conditions. The effect was more pronounced when all the stressors were applied in combination followed by performance under M, then T and N. All three stressors caused impaired dexterity and an increase in the incidence of errors.

An error that a surgeon makes can be categorised into two types: skill based or knowledge based. Skill-based errors involve, as in this experiment, dropped objects and objects placed incorrectly in the disc, while knowledge-based errors occurred when objects were placed in the wrong area. Both skill- and knowledge-based errors increased across all stress-inducing conditions. If there was one particular stressor that caused the most errors, it was the 'noise'. The fact that noise itself caused the maximum number of errors highlights the necessity to improve the environment in which surgeons perform. Admittedly, both types of errors increased under the effect of all stresses in combination;

however, skill-based errors increased by a much larger proportion than knowledge-based errors.

As compared with open surgery, video-assisted surgery is perceived to be more stressful and to involve a higher degree of concentration. Also, fatigue after performing these procedures due to inappropriate ergonomics is higher. Thus, it is possible that the impact of stress-inducing factors is more harmful in the case of video endoscopic tasks than it is in open procedures.

Surgical instrument stability is integral to surgical success, especially microsurgical success, and is largely influenced by hand tremor. Stress is known to worsen hand tremors. People drink coffee, tea or other stimulants that are known to affect hand tremors. When they are experiencing stress, they may consume these drinks more often. In the case of surgeons, they need to consider what effect it would have on dexterity. Although the detrimental effects of tremors are known, studies have not been done to determine the effect on microsurgical stability. To address this issue, a study was conducted to measure the effects of caffeine and propranolol on surgeons' hand tremors during simulated microsurgery.[5] The researchers objectively measured hand tremor following the administration of placebo, caffeine, or propranolol.

On three separate days, hand tremor was measured immediately before and one hour after ingestion of placebo, caffeine or propranolol. Tremors were measured using the Microsurgery Advanced Design Laboratory Stability, Activation, and Maneuverability tester (MADSAM). The MADSAM uses a magnetic field sensor and customised software to correlate magnetic field strength with physical location. The MADSAM can record the position of a microsurgical instrument at an accuracy of 1 micrometre.

The results showed that ingestion of caffeine increased mean tremor by 31% over baseline and propranolol reduced it by 22%. The largest increases in hand tremor within the caffeine group were from subjects who indicated no daily caffeine use. When propranolol was consumed, the results for blood pressure and pulse closely followed those of hand tremor measurement. Thus the results of performance tests following caffeine ingestion, combined with subjective interviews, suggest that individuals who do not regularly consume caffeinated products tend to respond adversely to caffeine.

Even though you may be convinced that stress affects surgeons' performance, the problem of identifying a surgeon who is stressed is a challenge. For some, the recognition of severe stress is dramatic and unquestioned. There are the tragic examples of surgeons who have committed suicide due to severe but unrecognised stress. Some have become entangled in the law because of driving under the influence, or being involved in accidents in which they were intoxicated. A surgeon who appears in the operating room intoxicated is very uncommon, but not unheard of.

Stress is often claimed by surgeons to be a precipitating factor for excessive alcohol consumption. However, this kind of behaviour may well compound poor performance and surgical errors and may in fact worsen the stress. Worsening of performance after being awake for 24 hours is comparable to the worsening of performance when your blood concentration of alcohol is 0.1%. Thus it would be helpful to examine the effects of alcohol on surgical performance in more detail. It is known that individuals underestimate the amount of alcohol they have consumed and its effect on performance. This tendency to underestimate is more relevant to the residual impairment after recovery from the alcohol. Societal norms forbid drinking in the hospital but are permissive of alcohol consumption during evenings prior to an operating day. Researchers decided to quantify the worsening of surgical performance over the course of a day following excessive alcohol consumption the previous evening.[6]

In the first part of the study, final-year students with no previous experience with the surgical simulator participated. In the second part, experienced surgeons participated. All participants completed a baseline trial on the simulator before consuming alcohol. All subjects were instructed to drink alcohol freely until they felt intoxicated. No doubt, the subjects thoroughly enjoyed participating in the study! Subjects were transported to the study laboratory at 8 a.m. the following morning and were tested at 9 a.m., 1 p.m. and 4 p.m. The outcome measures were time to task completion, mean errors and efficiency of instrument use.

Results showed that in the first part, alcohol-associated performance degradation was found in students who were intoxicated. The deterioration in performance lasted until 4 p.m. the following day. For the second part of the study, at 9 a.m. on the day after consumption of excess alcohol, the experts completed the task faster than they did during the baseline period.

However, by 1 p.m., they were performing significantly worse than at 9 a.m. Their performance returned to baseline levels by 4 p.m. Although by 4 p.m. their time to complete the task had returned to baseline, their error rate was higher and economy of movements was significantly worse throughout the following day. These differences occurred notwithstanding the extensive experience the surgeons had. One may wonder why the expert surgeons had unexpectedly faster completion time at 9 a.m. relative to the baseline. We need to be clear that time taken to complete the task is not a reliable parameter when taken in isolation. While it is possible that elements of either training effect or loss of inhibition may be contributory, when taken in combination with the significantly worsened error score and poor instrument efficiency, it cannot be taken as a marker of improved performance.

So far we have seen evidence that shows how operative stress and chemicals that are used to deal with the stress affect surgical performance. The evidence was obtained by employing various methods and experiments. However, simply asking surgeons what they think about the effect of stress on their performance can give interesting information. That is what was done in a qualitative study, mentioned earlier, which explored surgeons' perceptions of stress.[7] 'People under stress want to get a lot of things done in a short space of time and, consequently, the chances of getting things wrong are a lot higher,' said one surgeon. When asked directly, most surgeons were not keen to talk about their own experience of stress and brushed it off by saying, 'I've learned to deal with pretty much everything, so very little stresses me.' However, when asked if they had ever seen someone else stressed, surgeons were more forthcoming. About half of the surgeons said that a small amount of stress is beneficial in that it aids concentration. Beyond that initial amount, stress was thought to negatively affect performance. Surgeons suggested that their decision making is particularly vulnerable to stress: 'You lose focus, can't think straight, and usually the stressful moments are a time when you need to be thinking quickly and clearly.'

SUMMARY

While making the decision about the operative procedure, the only factors taken into consideration are the risk and benefits of the operation to the patient. Although it is intuitive that excessive levels of stress can affect performance, the level of stress experienced by the surgeon in a particular operation never arises as a potential contributor to outcome. Ascertaining the association between stress and performance is not easy. From the studies which have shown the association, the following themes emerge: a surgeon, especially an inexperienced one, performing a simple but novel task suffers stress to the degree that the quality of even basic skills is detrimentally affected. Both skill-based and knowledge-based skills are affected by stress. Better technical performance and strategies to mitigate the effects of stress are key skills in dealing with situations that are unavoidably stressful.

REFERENCES

1 Schwaitzberg S.D., Godinez C., Kavic S., Sutton E., et al. Training and working in high-stakes environments: lessons learned and problems shared by aviators and surgeons. *Surg Innov.* 2009: 16(2): 187–95.

2 Arora S., Sevdalis N., Aggarwal R., Sirimanna P., et al. Stress impairs psychomotor performance in novice laparoscopic surgeons. *Surg Endosc.* 2010; 24: 2588–93.

3 Schuetz M., Gockel I., Beardi J., Hakman P., et al. Three different types of surgeon-specific stress reactions identified by laparoscopic immolation in a virtual scenario. *Surg Endosc.* 2008; 22: 1263 7.

4 Moorthy K., Munz Y., Dosis A., Bann S., Darzi A. The effect of stress-inducing conditions on the performance of a laparoscopic task. *Surg Endosc.* 2003; 17: 1481–4.

5 Humayun M.U., Rader R.S., Pieramici D.J., Awh C.C., de Juan E. Jr. Quantitative measurement of the effects of caffeine and propranolol on surgeon hand tremor. *Arch Ophthalmol.* 1997; 115(3): 371–4.

6 Gallagher A.G., Boyle E., Toner P., Neary P.C., et al. Persistent next-day effects of excessive alcohol consumption on laparoscopic surgical performance. *Arch Surg.* 2011; 146(4): 419–26.

7 Arora S., Sevdalis N., Nestel D., Tierney T., et al. Managing intraoperative stress: what do surgeons want from a crisis training program? *Am J Surgery.* 2009; 197: 537–43.

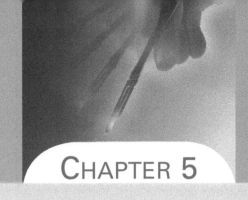

CHAPTER 5

What stresses surgeons?

Acknowledging the stress surgeons experience in the operation room was the initial step in addressing the issue. The next step was to find out if it does have any impact on surgical performance. Since we have explored both these steps, we now need to focus on finding out what specific factors contribute to the stress. This is a multifactorial issue, so we will have to look at a range of elements.

Surgeons are exposed to significant stress-inducing conditions in the operating room. It could be a residual stress due to a critically ill patient in the HDU or an administrative workload. Surgeons often are under time pressure because of scheduling problems and excessive workload. Noise is rife in all operating theatres, which sometimes have been equated to 'freeways'. The noise levels can be as high as 80 to 100 dB. Such high levels of noise are harmful to the performance and an obstruction to communication. These stress-inducing conditions frequently intermix rather than occurring as isolated events.

There is a view that video-assisted surgery requires more concentration than open surgery and that the instrument and visual difficulties make it more stressful. Cuschieri described a 'surgical fatigue syndrome' that occurs after performing endoscopic surgery for more than four hours.[1] A study confirmed that endoscopic surgery is more stressful than open surgery.[2]

A workstation was created to compare the mental workload of surgeons. The surgeons, from various experience levels, were asked to do endoscopic knot tying. The level of stress was assessed in three ways: subjective reports of stress; tonic skin conductance level (SCL); and electro-oculogram. The frequency of the eye blink as picked up by electro-oculogram is a measure of mental load. Eye-blink rate is affected by both degree of mental concentration and the perceived stress. The surgeons were assessed in three different conditions: resting condition; open technique; and endoscopic technique.

Frequency of eye blinks decreased when surgeons performed an open surgical task from a resting condition. This was due to the surgeon's increased level of mental concentration. When the task changed from open to endoscopic, the frequency of eye blinks increased. The increase in the eye-blink rate from open to endoscopic task is consistent with the high demand level relative to open surgery. It is decreased by increased concentration and increased by increased task demand. So one can see a U-shaped eye-blink response.

It was also seen that surgeons tied fewer knots using the endoscopic technique than when using the open technique. The decreased number of knots was thought to be due to deterioration in performance. The third parameter, skin conductance, increased progressively from rest to the open task and then to the endoscopic task. It also correlated with the subjective increase in stress perception. Experienced surgeons showed less variability in SCL across tasks. SCL is known to increase with stress level and the increase is known to correlate with myocardial activity. The correlation between the SCL recordings, surgeon's performance and subjective self-assessments, taken together, strengthens the perception that endoscopic surgery requires greater concentration and places greater mental stress on surgeons than the same procedure done by open technique.

If you look at the various untoward surgical events, you may agree that, in the hospital, the operating room is the most likely place for an error to occur. Many of the errors occur due to working with uncertainty in the situations where too many demands and conflicting priorities need to be managed. Besides, many operating suites are designed in such a way that they are not fit for the present purpose. Every day new technologies are introduced, working teams keep on changing and within this unsettling working environment, a surgeon is expected to perform under substantial pressure in a precise manner. If you separate these factors and see the impact of each independently, it may be minimal, but when seen collectively, they can lead to serious human failure. The situation can be described as 'death by a thousand paper cuts'. One of such factors, one of the thousand paper cuts that cause the surgeon to become stressed, is ergonomics in the operating theatre.

Dr Berguer, a chief of surgery in California, remembers his residency days when laparoscopic surgical procedures were introduced. As he began performing increasingly complex laparoscopic procedures, he started experiencing pain in his upper body after he left the operating room. He realised that as a surgeon he depended on tools to conduct his trade and how he works with these tools affected not only the clinical outcome but also his own health.[2] While performing minimal invasive surgery, surgeons hold instruments in unsupported positions, and after chronic stress the effects of the wear and tear become apparent. Dr Berguer came to know of surgeons who suffered upper limb muscle injuries and had to stay away from surgery for some time due to this occupational stress.

Any surgical procedure requires standing, awkward body positions, and the need to exert force. However, surgeons performing video-assisted procedures move around less than during open surgery and hold body postures longer, increasing their physical fatigue.[3] These issues like awkward positions while operating and the placement of the operating table and monitor add to the stress. The resulting pain and stiffness that surgeons experience after operations add to the psychological toll.

Initial surveys identifying ergonomic problems showed that up to 30% of surgeons experienced them. But recent surveys showed that up to 90% of responding surgeons had physical discomfort attributable to performing minimal invasive surgery.[4] The impact of ergonomic factors may surprise some surgeons, especially those who are still young. Dr Adrian Park, a general surgeon in the USA, participated in an ergonomic experiment when he was in his thirties, conducted by an industrial ergonomics group. The study tested the impact of endoscopic surgery on the surgeon's body. As Dr Park performed a routine procedure that took him less than 25 minutes to complete, the researchers studied the biomechanics of his movements. Dr Park was astounded when the researcher told him that if he were an industrial business, they would have to shut him down! The results revealed many ergonomic risk factors that violated industrial standards. Specifically, it was noted that movements involved with the endoscopic procedure had significant biomechanical impact mirrored by muscle strain, sustained contraction and excessive joint deflection.[5]

Many of the studies that have explored surgeons' stress have been carried out in laboratory settings. This laboratory setting may not be representative of and generalisable to real operating rooms. Studies that have used real operating rooms have used observational techniques by focusing on problems in one specific domain or one stress-inducing factor. In addition to biases discussed earlier, these studies are likely to undervalue the impact of stress because of reluctance among surgeons to accept that stress is a part of practice. There is little evidence thus far on the bigger picture that quantifies the true incidence of stressors in surgery as they occur in real time and compares them with surgeons' own self-perceptions.

A study aimed to fill this gap was carried out.[6] This was an observational study to quantify factors causing stress in the operating room and their incidence. The information was collected while the operations were performed in 55 elective procedures.

A wide variety of cases were included, such as hernias, appendectomies, laparoscopic cholecystectomies, and total hip replacements. The duration of observation varied from 15 minutes for the case of examination under anaesthesia to 8 hours for an oesophagectomy. During each case, one observer recorded activities and events that occurred by using what is known as 'ethnographic field note' techniques. Recorded observations included occurrences such as communications between the surgeon and other team members, entrances and exits of individuals, surgical events, and distractions such as background noise.

To determine each surgeon's perceived stress levels, surgeons were asked to report their level of stress during the surgery. The State Trait Anxiety Inventory (STAI), which quantifies different aspects of stress, was used.

Surgeons were asked to rate how stressful they found eight specific factors during the procedure on a scale of 1 to 10 (1 not stressful at all; 10 extremely stressful), which was called the Surgical Environment Assessment (SEA) score.

The factors in SEA included:

1. Technical problems
2. Patient problems
3. Teamwork problems
4. Time and management issues

5. Distractions/interruptions
6. Equipment problems
7. Personal problems
8. Teaching a junior colleague.

The ratings across these eight factors were subsequently summed to give a global score of stress in the surgical environment for each case: minimum score, 8; maximum score, 80. The observer was also asked to rate similarly on these factors. This SEA score was then correlated with the surgeons' STAI score (minimum score 6; maximum score 24) to determine if self-reported stress levels were a function of the surgical stressors present in the environment.

The investigators found that a total of 323 factors or incidences as potential stressors were identified across 55 cases, with the average frequency of six stressors per case. This confirms the array of stressors that surgeons face in the operating room; also it gives us quantified incidence of these stressors. Self-reported stress scores confirmed that at times surgeons experience extremely high levels of stress. Some stressors occur frequently but are not significant while others are infrequent but have significant impact. Among the various factors, the stress caused by technical factors had the highest impact.

Another study observed the operating room environment but the researchers did not focus their observation only on surgeons.[7] They saw the impact of distractions and interruptions on surgeons, anaesthetists, and nurses during routine surgical procedures. The operating room staff experienced disruptions in 33% to 47% of the procedures. Other investigators have noted similar frequency of distractions; an average of 13 distracting events per procedure. Interestingly, the surgeons in this study perceived significantly fewer disruptions than the anaesthetic or nursing staff. The overall disruptions rate was reported to be 25% by surgeons, 37% by anaesthetists, and 42% by nurses.

Among the distractions and interruptions, those related to equipment, communication, and the operative environments occurred most commonly and were most visibly disruptive. People coming into and leaving the operating room frequently cause significant distractions. Those visitors who interact with surgeons are less distracting than those interacting with nurses or anaesthetists. Frivolous background conversations (small talk) may help reduce the stress and tensions of the operating team but may also be more distracting than quieter, non-describable noise. The most distracting communications were those related to operating room equipment and provisions, responses to queries about other patients, ongoing management of the operating list with the members of the operating room team, and teaching that surgeons had to deliver as they were performing.

Based on research and personal experience, the researchers developed the Disruptions in Surgery Index (DiSI).

DiSI score = Disruption Frequency × Disruption severity

This means that each disruption can be characterised for frequency and severity. A high DiSI score can be a function of an accumulation of many low-disruptive events (e.g. bleeps) or few really disruptive events (e.g. unavailable test result). The total score provides an indication of the total amount of disruption, which can then be examined for high-frequency/low-severity events, and/or low-frequency/high-severity events.

Surgical disruptions can be categorised into seven domains:

1. **Individuals' personality:** evidence suggests that personality characteristics affect teamwork in operating rooms.[8]
2. **Operating room environment:** this relates to the environmental conditions of an operating room and the distractions obtained in the observational studies (bleeps, phone calls, unavailable equipment, door-openings etc.).
3. **Communication:** inclusion of communication as a separate disruption type was informed by the presence of communication as a major dimension in surgical teamwork.
4. **Coordination and situational awareness:** e.g. managing the operating lists during the course of the day, people being late or absent.
5. **Patient-related disruptions:** this disruption touches on a major patient safety issue.
6. **Team cohesion:** this reflects individual team members feeling part of and identifying with the team.
7. **Organisational disruptions:** these encapsulate some of the macro-management issues that affect working in an operating room, including the fact that the delivery of surgical services and teaching

occur concurrently and under time pressure (because of staffing levels, waiting lists, etc.). Some of these issues appeared in our observational studies.

The qualitative study, mentioned earlier, that explored surgeons' perceptions of key surgical stresses, was able to elaborate on the stressors further.[9] Interviews elucidated the following sources of stress:

1. Emergency cases
2. Surgical complications
   Surgical error
   Unexpected bleeding
   Difficulties in finding the source of a problem
   No progress
3. Advanced tasks
   Complex procedure
   High-risk patient
   Multitasking
   Time pressure
   Immediate decision making
4. Equipment problems
   Missing equipment
   Equipment failure
   Unfamiliar equipment
5. Teamwork problems
   Incompetent staff
   Inexperienced staff
   Language problems
   Staff not paying attention
   Interpersonal issues
6. Distractions
   Talking noises
   People walking in and out
   Bleeps
   Phone calls

7. Personal factors

Tiredness

Hunger

Illness

Physical discomfort

Personal problems.

Stress during operating procedure is seen in emergency cases as well as elective operations. Apart from obvious clinical differences, the demands placed on the operating surgeon are also quite different. For example, the team members involved in an elective surgery are usually constant and there is familiarity and certainty with the operative team. On the other hand, in the case of an emergency procedure, there may not exist any familiarity or understanding between the surgeon and other members. This situation places additional demand on surgeons' stress-management skills. They have to place different emphasis in the two different situations. Since it is assumed that the stress during elective surgery is less than during the emergency surgery, the frequency of intraoperative errors is likely to be less. Ironically, studies have observed the opposite; the likelihood of an error is higher in an elective case than in an emergency. This could be due to the fact of reduced alertness and being presumptuous. Errors are more often to lack of diligence and not implementing ordinary skills rather than to lack of extraordinary skills. Elective procedures are scheduled after consideration of clinical details and appropriate preparation. This may cause the surgeon to become 'off guard' and get caught in an unanticipated problem. When you are not prepared, alertness is reduced and the thought process shifts into automatic mode. You may miss some cues that would have warned you of an impending problem.

SUMMARY

Surgeons are exposed to a range of considerable stress-inducing conditions while performing procedures. If one looks at the impact of each of these conditions independently, it may be minimal, but when seen collectively, they can lead to a serious human failure. The situation can be described as 'death by a thousand paper cuts'. Potential stressors include operating itself as compared to ward work, and being the primary operator as compared to assisting the operation. Video endoscopic surgery is a common potential stressor compared with open surgery. Other stressors include complexity of a procedure, intraoperative bleeding, and equipment problems. Non-technical sources of stress include distractions, time pressure, being on call, external visitors in the operating room, and having the operation being broadcast live. Experience seems to moderate stress levels, with seniors seemingly better adapted to stressful situations.

REFERENCES

1 Cuschieri A. Whither minimal access surgery: tribulations and expectations. *Am J Surg.* 1995; 169: 9–19.

2 Berguer R., Smith W.D., Chung Y.H. Performing laparoscopic surgery is significantly more stressful for the surgeon than open surgery. *Surg Endosc.* 2001; 15: 1204–7.

3 Glickson J. Surgeons experience more ergonomic stress in the OR. *Bull Am Coll Surg.* 2012; 97(4): 20–6.

4 Nguyen N.T., Ho H.S., Smith W.D., Philipps C., et al. An ergonomic evaluation of surgeons' axial skeletal and upper extremity movements during laparoscopic and open surgery. *Am J Surg.* 2010; 182(6): 720–4.

5 Park A., Lee G., Seagull F.J., Meenaghan N., Dexter D. Patients benefit while surgeons suffer: an impending epidemic. *J Am Coll Surg.* 2010; 210(3): 306–13.

6 Arora S., Hull L., Sevdalis N., Tierney T., et al. Factors compromising safety in surgery: stressful events in the operating room. *Am J Surg.* 2010; 199: 60–5.

7 Sevdalis N., Forrest D., Undre S., Darzi A., Vincent C. Annoyances, disruptions, and interruptions in surgery: the Disruptions in Surgery Index (DiSI). *World J Surg.* 2008; 32: 1643–50.

8 Katz J.D. Conflict and its resolution in the operating room. *J Clin Anesth.* 2007; 19: 152–8.

9 Wetzel C.M., Kneebone R.L., Wolosynowych M., Nestel D., et al. The effects of stress on surgical performance. *Am J Surg.* 2006; 191: 5–10.

Chapter 6

Situation awareness and stress in surgery

Situation awareness is remaining alert in order to maintain presence of mind during an operative procedure. In other words, it is a mental state in which you are fully aware of your actions and their effects and have a plan if you need to make changes in your actions. If we think about professionals who need to be extremely vigilant about their surroundings while carrying out their work, we can't think of anybody other than soldiers. In the battlefield, unless soldiers remain fully alert, it may cost them their lives. No wonder the concept of situation awareness was first introduced in the military. Having considered the concept and its application, one can appreciate that it is also valid in the operating theatre. Due to lack of situation awareness, soldiers have lost their lives, and patients have lost their lives when surgeons overlooked it in an operating room. Soldiers are supposed to be aware of the battlefield and the enemy position before the enemy becomes aware of theirs. Surgeons need to maintain awareness of the operative field and the likely consequences of their actions before a disaster strikes. Thus it involves keeping an eye on the operative field, especially on crucial anatomical structures, finding out if there is any change in respect of physiology or pathology and predicting immediate steps to be taken.

The term 'situation awareness' may be new in surgery but the situations that ensue from lack of awareness must be familiar: not being aware that a patient has lost too much blood and is hypovolaemic; or having cut a nerve that was supposed to be preserved to maintain vital function. These incidences reflect loss of situation awareness. When a surgeon says something like 'Oh, I didn't realise …' or 'To be honest, I wasn't aware …' one can expect that the problem must have occurred due to loss of situation awareness.

Way and his colleagues analysed 252 cases of laparoscopic bile duct injuries. They found that 97% of cases happened due to loss of situation awareness rather than technical issues. Specifically, the problems were related to reception and interpretation of visual information. In 22% of cases the procedure was routine and in 75% of cases the surgeon did not even realise that the bile duct had been cut; thus offering further evidence of losing situation awareness.[1] Dekker and Hugh studied loss of situation awareness in 42 bile duct injury cases from the psychological perspective.[2] They concluded that one of the problems in those cases was underestimation of the risk and not interpreting the visual information. Although the visual information was ambiguous and should have been challenged by the surgeon, she went ahead by accepting it. She did not give it a second thought, which she would have if she had maintained situation awareness.

Cases have happened in the operating room where situation awareness got lost due a simple action like not placing the X-ray appropriately on the viewer. A child was taken to the operating theatre to have a chest drain inserted for pneumothorax. To decide which side the drain needed to be put in, the surgeon asked for the chest X-ray to be shown on the viewer. Looking at the X-ray, he decided the drain needed to go in the right side. After the procedure, when a follow-up X-ray was taken, it showed the pneumothorax on the opposite side and not on the side where the drain was inserted. How did it happen? It became apparent that before the drain was inserted, when the X-ray was shown on the viewer, the sides got flipped; the right side was seen on the left and the left was seen on the right. Due to the pneumothorax on the left side, the heart was pushed to the right, thus, although the X-ray viewing had switched the sides, nobody noticed it. Since nobody checked if the X-ray had been correctly shown, the visual impression was taken for granted and a decision was made.[3]

Maintaining situation awareness is a three-step process. It starts with information gathering about the existing situation, interpreting the information from other available sources and using knowledge and experience to make sense of the information to take appropriate action.

1. **Gathering information.** While performing the procedure, you receive information from various sources: anatomical information from the operating field, monitors informing you about physiological parameters, and other team members such as an anaesthetist who will tell you of any changes in clinical status. Sometimes there is so much information that it is difficult to prioritise. In stressful situations, some relevant information may get overlooked.

2. **Interpreting the information.** There is no point in obtaining information if you are unable to understand and interpret it in the prevailing context. This is where experience comes into play. If you do not have the knowledge or experience, although the information may be there, you will not appreciate its significance. A problem is seen in a case where information received is expected to change the course of the procedure. However, the surgeon decides to carry on without making any changes in the plan. This happens because of confirmation bias – a cognitive error in which the individual sticks to the plan in spite of the situation having changed and information suggesting that the plan needs to change.

3. **Anticipation and preparation.** Experienced surgeons take the recent information into consideration and prepare for a future course. This may or may not involve a change of plan. If they have any doubt or uncertainty, they discuss with other team members for clarification.

Here are two examples of a progression of a case and changes in situation awareness.

A surgeon decided to perform video-assisted adrenalectomy. She mulled over whether the procedure needed to be done by open approach or whether it was safe to do it endoscopically. At the beginning of the procedure, she thought she would be able to do it endoscopically. However, during the procedure the patient's blood pressure started falling. It became apparent that the patient was bleeding from somewhere and the source could not be seen with the endoscope. With this new information she decided to abandon the endoscopic procedure and switch to an open procedure. The source of the bleeding was found and was ameliorated. The rest of the procedure and the recovery were uneventful.

In another case, the surgeon observed that there was too much bleeding in the operative field (perceiving the information). Having ruled out other causes of excessive bleeding, he started wondering if the patient had developed coagulopathy (interpreting the information).

He decided that it was technically difficult to repair the tear in a conventional way and decided to use glue before going ahead (projection and anticipation).

Let us look at the above three stages in further detail.

1. INFORMATION GATHERING

For gathering information we use various senses, from visual to olfactory. The perception of visual information is obvious: the operating field and the anatomical details we perceive visually. If it is a video-assisted procedure, the TV monitor gives you an idea about the placement of an instrument. We also observe the behaviour and actions of the assisting surgeon. The tactile sense gives information about the texture of the tissue and tension of the sutures. Kinaesthetic sense makes us aware of gross and fine movements. If you are performing an intestinal surgery and you start smelling faecal matter, you get concerned about a bowel injury. The auditory signals from monitors or a comment from an assistant or the anaesthetist give you an update on the patient through the auditory modality. Thus information to maintain situation awareness is received all the time and from various modalities. Whether the surgeon is able to pick up this information and take it to the next stage depends on alertness, level of distractions in the room, level of motivation and the degree of stress.

We do come across surgeons who have developed good habits of gathering the information effectively. If you observe these surgeons, you notice that they diligently carry out preoperative checks of a patient's details, confirm that all the necessary investigations have been carried out and that the results are available to them. They also maintain good rapport with team members, especially the anaesthetists. Since they are acutely aware of the information they would need from monitors and other equipment, they carefully align the equipment including operation table and lights according to the type of the procedure and their own preference. During the procedure you can see them actively updating the information by watching the monitors or asking the anaesthetist for the update.

On the other hand, there are surgeons who lose situation awareness from the first step. These are the surgeons who hurriedly enter the operating room, do not show any concern for whether the relevant investigations have been done, and if they have been, whether the results are available to them in the operating room. It is a common scenario to see surgeons in the middle of the surgery asking somebody to get hold of the clinical notes and request them to read out either a result of the investigation they had done in the past or some clinical plan written by them. They are usually known for not maintaining good rapport with the nurses and anaesthetist, thereby compromising important sources of information. This scenario is particularly common among surgeons who have an overbooked surgical schedule with multiple cases and who have to switch from one operating room to another to complete their scheduled cases on time. When the surgeon is rushing from one case to the other, there is little time for information gathering and even less time to process the available information.

It was not uncommon for Dr MS, an orthopaedic surgeon in the USA, to schedule multiple spine surgeries back to back on his operating days. Indeed, he was a busy surgeon and it only made sense for him to schedule as many cases as possible to be efficient and productive. In addition, being in private practice, there was the issue of declining revenue due to decreased reimbursements from the health insurance companies and increasing overhead expenses. It was not easy being an orthopaedic surgeon in private practice, what with the rapid changes in the healthcare environment. On one such busy operating day, he was about to operate on one of his patients who had a lumbar disc prolapse with radiating pain in the right lower extremity. He was in a particular rush on this day, as he was already running behind on his schedule of surgeries. His previous surgery had run over time due to an unexpected complication that was encountered intraoperatively. Upon completion of the procedure, he had barely any time to enter postoperative physician orders and for the postoperative conference with the anxious family members of this patient. Thereafter, he walked over briskly to the preoperative patient holding area and as usual he met with the next patient and the family members. He quickly confirmed the symptoms of pain, paraesthesia and weakness to be in the right lower extremity, and, as per the checklist protocol, he marked his initials on the surgical site with indelible ink. The patient was then wheeled into the operating room and was positioned, prepped and draped under his supervision. During 'time-out', the operating room staff member appropriately mentioned the name of the patient, the diagnosis, and planned procedure to treat the lumbar disc prolapse on the right side of the patient. Dr MS then made the incision through the skin and the fascia and dissected down to the lumbar disc level and to his surprise there was no evidence of a disc prolapse despite extensive search for one. He then confirmed the lumbar vertebral level to be correct by analysing the preoperative imaging studies. By now he was sweating and nervous and cursing his luck for having such a stressful day. Pacing back to the patient, he immediately realised his mistake. He had inadvertently made the incision on the left side instead of on the right side of the spine.

Surgeons who are able to maintain situation awareness develop the sensitivity to notice (apparently) minor cues and incongruities even in a routine case. This has been recognised as one of the features of expertise. This is not to say that they never have difficulties with situation awareness. At times there are valid reasons for the surgeon to experience problems in maintaining situation awareness. There are various factors that cause difficulty in gathering information. Appearance or presentation of the information is so inconspicuous that it may be difficult to notice it even for an expert. In other cases, the information may not be present, or there may be changes in the patient's status since the procedure began. And there are well-documented cases that show the incidences of misperception.

It is a common observation that we miss information in stressful situations. It can happen due to what is called 'tunnel vision'. In this situation your perception narrows down so much that your attention is focused on a very limited part of the procedure. In a well-known case of an elective nasal surgery, the anaesthetist tried to intubate the patient but failed even after repeated attempts. Everybody in the operating room became stressed and focused their attention on exploring different ways to intubate the patient. They became so engrossed in trying to intubate that they were not able to pick up the hypoxic status that became seriously low. If they had noticed the hypoxia in time, alternative measures such as a tracheostomy could have taken place. Unfortunately, the patient died due to cerebral hypoxia.[4] There are incidences where surgeons did not notice the amount of blood loss while their attention was focused on finding the source of bleeding. Due to tunnel vision they failed to register the duration and quantity of blood loss. A surgeon who has situation awareness would do it differently. Instead of continuing frantic efforts to find the bleeder, she would apply pressure with packs and, while maintaining the pressure, try to assess the amount of blood loss and take the necessary measures. Some surgeons lose their attention very easily and take their eyes off the case as they start thinking about some other matter to do with the patient.

The fallibility of sensory and memory systems gets exposed in stressful situations. One specific type of weakness is 'change blindness'. In this case, people fail to realise the key element they were expected to observe has changed while they have been monitoring the situation.

A research experiment was conducted to assess the effect of change blindness. On a busy road of a metropolitan city centre, a person, chosen randomly from the street, was asked for directions by an investigator. The person started telling him how to reach the destination. While the person was giving the direction another person carrying a huge wooden board walked between the two people in such a way that both the persons, one giving the direction and the investigator, could not see each other for few seconds. During this brief period of a few seconds, researchers replaced the investigator who asked for the directions. They wanted to find out if the person giving the direction was able to recognise that the individual had changed. Interestingly, half of the individuals giving directions did not notice the change and continued giving directions where they left off before the interruption.[5]

You may experience this kind of situation in endoscopic surgery where the area under vision is small. When you move away from the main area to release some tissue and then resume the dissection, you may overlook some changes that may have occurred when you moved away.

It is also a common experience that when we are deeply involved in a particular task we miss auditory stimuli like a doorbell or phone ringing. This type of attention problem is called inattention deafness. When you are engrossed in the procedure there is a possibility that you may miss verbal information given to you by an assistant or a nurse. Problems of attention do not necessarily occur due to distracting external stimuli; they can occur otherwise. In a protracted case where the assistant has been holding a retractor and is not much interested in this tedious procedure, the assistant is likely to drift into inner thought processes and lose attention. This is seen to happen with anaesthetists as well.

2.   UNDERSTANDING AND INTERPRETING THE INFORMATION

If you hear a change in the monitor sound or observe changes in the tracing while operating, you have only cleared the first step in maintaining situation awareness. The next step is to understand and interpret that information. The changes in the monitor signals may indicate some anaesthetic problem, or it may be some technical matter with the sensors, or it may be due to your handling of a particular tissue like the vagus nerve or a carotid body. If the changes are the result of your actions, you need to understand the consequences. For example, whether the patient is likely to have bradycardia or the rhythm is going to return to normality soon. Once new clinical information is received, we check its relevance with the knowledge we have in long-term memory. With experience we create patterns of clinical situations. We match the newly received information with that pattern and make sense of it. This happens automatically without any active effort on our part. Thus there is very little use of conscious memory, provided you have patterns in your long-term memory. Although this automatic process saves conscious working memory, it is not without problems. Being automatic, this process takes place without any scrutiny of the information. It is as if, when your car approaches the gate, the barrier is lifted automatically without checking entry permits for your car. Our perception may be distorted or may not be appropriate in the existing context. Due to the automaticity we may come to a wrong conclusion. The study described earlier about injury to the bile duct describes how the surgeon did not realise the injury due to misperception.

Experienced surgeons don't rely on a single source of information; they have skills to recognise and understand information from various sources like operative field, monitors, actions by the anaesthetist and so on. When you have started performing laparoscopic cholecystectomy and, after inflating the abdomen, you see the anaesthetist picking up an atropine ampule, you would assume that the patient has bradycardia. You will look at the monitor and confirm your interpretation of the situation. Because of your knowledge and past experience, you will conclude that the bradycardia is the result of increased intra-abdominal pressure caused by the inflation. This process of receiving and interpreting the information is supported by the patterns or mental models about the clinical situations we already have in our memory.

Surgeons who are successful in maintaining situation awareness are usually good at analysing the information gathered from preoperative investigations and the operative findings in front of them. While operating, they continue to check if there is any variation between the preoperative investigations and operative findings. If they do find any variation, they will make an attempt to explain the disparity and will evaluate its significance.

On the other hand, surgeons who deviate from maintaining situation awareness are likely to miss a significant finding in the preoperative investigations. While performing the procedure, they appear to be struggling with what they see in the operative field. Some surgeons are in the habit of verbalising their thoughts. The kind of question surgeons raise would give an observer an idea of the lack of understanding they have about the pathology or the nature of problem and their expectations of outcome. Moreover, rather than seeking clarification about some information that does not fit their pattern, they are quick to discard it, concluding that it is not relevant. These are the kind of warning signals indicating an impending crisis in the procedure.

If the information you are getting does not match the pattern, you will have to bring it back to working memory and think about it consciously. This happens when you have come across an anatomical variant that you have never seen before. In this situation you will consciously think about various alternatives or may like to seek more information such as ordering a radiological investigation on the table.

The more patterns you have in your memory, the easier it will be for the information to get matched. If you have fewer patterns, as happens with inexperienced surgeons, you will have to keep the information in working memory. For the processing of the new information you will need to create a new pattern. In this kind of situation, the inexperienced surgeon will seek advice from an experienced surgeon who already has more patterns in stock. For this reason, when experienced surgeons operate, they appear to be good at recognising potential disaster early in the case before anyone else notices it. Not only are they able to recognise the impending problem, they also know the specific consequences if the problem is not dealt with appropriately. It is as if they have a whole plan of the operation with different trajectories and as soon as they see even a minor deviation from the plan, they are able to fast-forward the scenarios in their mind, which tells them where it will end up if things are not brought back on track.

One may get an impression that bringing new information into long-term memory is the only way to check the relevance of new information. It is not so. Surgeons also use patterns or mental models continuously as a method of ongoing surveillance during the operation. This is like closed-circuit TV cameras monitoring the activity at the security gates continuously. As soon as some unusual activity is noticed, the security staff are alerted. So what happens when a surgeon divides a nerve that is supposed to be preserved or nicks an artery that is not supposed to be touched? This can happen even though the surgeon has good ana-tomical understanding. This happens where mental models create an expectation and you adjust the information to fit the expectation. In other cases, it can happen that correct information is checked with an incorrect mental model and thus no abnormality is found.

In addition to existing mental models in stock, we also prepare new models or adjust existing ones just before we start the procedure. This adjustment is based upon preoperative investigations. To make correct adjustments and avoid missing any relevant information, a surgical checklist is used. This is aimed at identifying and avoiding any risk. However, if it is not implemented in its true spirit, and is carried out only as a tick-box exercise, specific information will be missed and the incorrect mental model will be activated.

Expert surgeons have more patterns in their head and not only do they adjust the pattern just before starting the procedure, but the adjustment is an ongoing process throughout the performance of the surgery. You cannot just discard the information if it doesn't fit into the existing pat-tern; you need to adjust the mental model accordingly. If that doesn't happen, you will fall into the trap of confirmation bias. You will accept only the information that fits into the existing mental model, discarding information that does not agree with it.

Conformation bias is more likely to happen in situations where the new information, if accepted, will involve additional effort. It is also likely to happen if the information indicates negative consequences. By their nature, surgeons are optimistic; hence they are likely to discard nega-tive information thinking that it is inconsequential. If the procedure has been more complex than you expected and has already exceeded the expected timeframe, and the new pathology you have found is likely to add work for which you were not prepared, it is likely to affect your thinking by adopting 'confirmation bias'. This kind of thinking is evident in situations where the surgeon is about to complete intestinal anastomosis in a procedure that has taken too long. Just after the last stitch the assistant informs the surgeon that he has noticed the colour of intestine becoming dusky. In this case, ideally, all stitches may need to come out and the anastomosis may need to be redone. The surgeon has two choices, either to spend some more time at the end of an arduous case when everybody is exhausted and redo the anastomosis, or to conclude that she has seen this kind of duskiness many times before without any consequences, and close the abdomen. The surgeon opting for the second choice indicates influence of confirmation bias. She is likely to learn the consequences of failing to pay heed to the information during the operation that would ask for adjustment in the mental model.

During this second step of situation awareness, problems can arise for various reasons. The problem may occur due to the surgeon not having a sufficient number of mental models as a result of inadequate experience. Even if there are sufficient models, the surgeon may choose a mental model that is not suitable for the existing case.

3. ANTICIPATING FUTURE EVENTS

The third and final step in maintaining situation awareness is anticipating what might happen next. You have received the information, you have checked the information with the knowledge and experience you have, now is the time to estimate future steps by combining past and present information. Anticipation involves predicting what may happen during the operation, specifically, as a result of the surgeon's actions. The prediction should also include events that could happen irrespective of his actions. The estimation could be as straightforward as estimating the size of prosthesis or any other implant that is going to be used in this case. In this step you mentally simulate future happenings and prepare for that eventuality. This way you are able to avoid any surprises. When you anticipate, it is likely to keep you alert. When you are anticipating that a major vessel is going to be near your area of dissection, you are going to be more vigilant. The expectancies you create are likely to enhance perception by focusing your attention. On the other hand, there is the potential of ignoring or misinterpreting the unexpected. Because you are confident about the anticipated events, if your focus of attention is too narrow, you may miss information that is beyond your circle of attention and is unexpected.

The behaviour of surgeons who are in the habit of anticipating events can be evident by their actions. They plan the operation list by taking into account potential delays. These delays may be due to surgical reasons or to other team members; for example, a particular anaesthetist taking a longer time to induce the patient. The surgeons not only plan the list, but also inform the staff of their needs in terms of instruments or equipment so that these are available when required. They appear clear in their messages or information and make the team members aware of contingency plans in case the current strategy fails.

We do notice the behaviour of surgeons who are known for 'losing the plot' during the procedure. They hardly discuss their plans with any other member in the team (maybe due to the fact that they may not have plans at all!). Their actions display overconfidence or disregard for what may go wrong. They are the kind of surgeon who underestimate blood loss in an elective procedure and for whose cases the anaesthetist remains extra cautious by keeping blood ready for transfusion without asking the surgeon. In the past such anaesthetists had to make frantic last-minute efforts to arrange for the blood since the surgeon was confident of 'not needing it'. These are the surgeons who, rather than anticipating a potential problem, wait for the problem to occur and then spend time and energy in 'firefighting'. Their colleagues question their judgements about operating on a particular patient when they would have sent the patient to a tertiary unit or to an expert who is known to operate on those types of cases routinely.

Maintaining situation awareness is particularly important for trainee surgeons. Failure to become situationally aware could be due to not having a mental model or simply not thinking far enough ahead from the present position (Figure 6.1). One can see indications of losing situation awareness among these inexperienced surgeons. To start with, they show a lack of required information, be it the investigations that they are supposed to have ready before the procedure or not being aware of the specific anatomical details of the patient. While performing an operation, they are expected to keep an eye on vital parameters like blood loss, which they fail to do. Everyone is aware that trainees take longer to perform a procedure; nevertheless, they frequently fail to perform the procedure in the time expected for an average trainee. They are in the habit of focusing attention on one thing by ignoring other equally relevant matters. You can see them complaining or spending too much time raising an equipment issue and not being attentive to the operative field. They exhibit inability to handle information coming from two different sources when the two pieces of information do not match each other. They get stuck when they come across what looks like the ureter but it does not vermiculate.

MEMORY SYSTEM AND SITUATION AWARENESS

In relation to situation awareness two types of memory systems are relevant. One is working memory or short-term memory and the second is long-term memory. Working memory has very limited capacity and it operates in conscious awareness. In stressful situations it is necessary to hold important information in working memory. One factor about working memory that is important in stressful situations is the fragility of that system. Being fragile, it becomes difficult to access the information in stressful periods. That is why some people becomes confused and behave haphazardly when under stress. In these situations, intensely concentrating on the task or repeating the information will help to access the information. Thus in an emergency situation, when every team member in the operating room is stressed, if you ask the nurse for a particular instrument, rather than getting frustrated for not getting the instrument, it is better to repeat the request since your initial request may have not gone into his working memory.

Because of limited capacity, working memory gets flooded with information very quickly. It is ideal if you are able to keep some spare capacity in working memory to deal with a sudden flux of information, especially in stressful situations. You may have observed that the operating surgeon asks for the music to be switched off as soon as he anticipates an impending problem. That way he can concentrate better and create room in working memory. Just like switching off music, you may consider any other activity that needs your conscious attention. If surgeons are not able to create space in working memory, they are unable to retrieve simple information like the names of the instrument they want from the nurse. When surgeons just raise their hand towards the nurse and are struggling to name the instrument (i.e. they develop nominal aphasia), assume that their working memory capacity has been exceeded and they need to offload some information. When you are thinking about the next steps of the procedure, you are employing working memory. In this situation a routine activity like even counting the swabs or instruments adds to the cognitive workload. Realising at

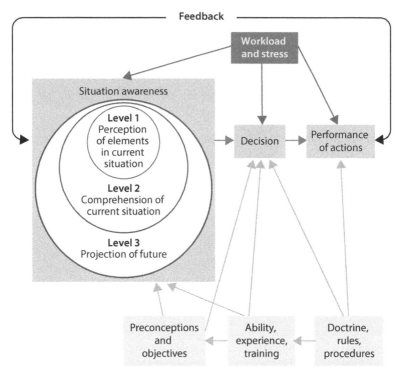

Figure 6.1 Model of situation awareness.

what time and in what way you can preserve the relevant information in working memory is important for maintaining situation awareness.

Long-term memory can store a huge amount of information that is acquired over the years. It is like a hard drive of a computer that can store many gigabytes of information. In that comparison, working memory capacity is like the storage capacity of a 10-year-old laptop. In the context of situation awareness, you retrieve the information from long-term memory, as needed, some of which is transferred temporarily to the working memory. You may have experienced that it is easier to recall certain types of information such as that which you have recently obtained or of a personal interest. After having returned from attending a workshop, it will be easier for you to apply the technique the following week for a similar patient since the technique is easier to pull into working memory.

FACTORS AFFECTING SITUATION AWARENESS

Stress and fatigue are important for their effect on situation awareness. Fatigue can be physical as well as mental. The fatigued brain loses capacity and speed in processing newly acquired information. It cannot hold the information in working memory for too long. This is one of the reasons behind exhausted doctors being prone to making more errors. Research has shown that reduction in a doctor's hours of work is associated with reduction in errors.[6]

The atmosphere in the operating room is bound to affect a team's situation awareness. If there is too much noise around, the surgeon may not be able to hear what is being said and may lose auditory information. This is especially relevant in operating rooms where loud music is played or various equipment is creating loud noise. Apart from noise, distractions such as phones ringing and movement of people do affect concentration. Due to such interruptions during a sequence of action, one has to 'back up' a few steps to regain the lost continuity.

To maintain situation awareness in the operating room surgeons may need to show leadership in controlling these environmental factors. They will have to make sure that nobody interrupts a team member, including themselves, during a task that requires use of working memory, such as a nurse counting swabs or instruments, or an anaesthetist checking drugs, etc. Trainees are more vulnerable than senior surgeons to the effect of distraction on situation awareness.

HOW TO MAINTAIN GOOD SITUATION AWARENESS

1. **Preoperative briefing:** If done appropriately, briefing will help the surgeon and others team members to understand the risk in the case. The concept of a WHO checklist that consists of introducing team members, explaining equipment requirements, clarifying patient's co-morbidities and verbalising anticipations works to achieve that aim.

2. **Mental preparation:** Systematic mental planning offers significant assistance in perception and anticipation once the procedure begins. This is described in detail in Chapter 9.

3. **Being fit for work:** Factors that affect the surgeon's well-being need to be addressed. Physical health issues like back pain or visual

difficulties affect capacity to concentrate and receive information respectively. Effect of alcohol is usually unrecognised but has noticeable impact.

4. **Managing distractions:** Although it may not be practical to keep the operating room 'distraction free' throughout the duration of the procedure, at least during a critical phase of the operation every effort should be made to achieve that. During take-off and landing of a plane, pilots maintain a 'sterile cockpit' – a concept that can be applied in the operating theatre. During critical phases of a flight, crew members are prohibited from carrying out any action that is non-essential and is likely to distract the pilot. Even the conversation between the professionals will be limited to the task at hand.

5. **Creating self-awareness:** Surgeons may inadvertently choose an inappropriate mental model to work with the received information. It is not easy to realise that the problem in the case resulted from the wrong mental model. Unless you regularly update and monitor your mental models about the specific procedure, you may never find the cause for 'losing the plot' frequently. It may be helpful to discuss your own perceptions of the situation with a colleague to have clarity about your interpretation. This is discussed in detail in Chapter 10.

6. **Involving other staff members:** Situation awareness is affected by other individuals in the operating room and the atmosphere, so it is not enough to rely solely on the surgeon to maintain it. Surgeons should encourage others to be proactive in giving them necessary information. If surgeons' attention is focused on the operative field, they are likely to miss information from the other side of the table. It is helpful for operating teams to have shared situation awareness.

7. **Avoid time pressure:** It is a matter of common sense to be aware that trying to finish the procedure hurriedly is not going to help situation awareness. This problem may occur due to improper planning of the operating list or by not anticipating the time needed for the major case. In several institutions, it is not uncommon for concurrent surgical procedures to be performed under the auspices of one attending or senior surgeon. The impact of such concurrent procedures on patient outcomes has yet to be fully investigated.

8. **Avoid over-delegating:** In some countries like the United States, there is an increasing trend of physician extenders and physician assistants being involved in the care of the patients. It is also not uncommon for the surgeon to rely more and more on the physician

assistant or nurse practitioner to collect and process information regarding the patient. This may result in a surgeon being poorly prepared for the surgical case due to inadequate information or poor processing of the information regarding the patient. While changes in healthcare economics and trends may be inevitable, a surgeon can avoid errors by being diligent about double-checking the information collected by the physician assistant or physician extender.

HOW TO FIND OUT IF YOU HAVE SITUATION AWARENESS

You may have come across a scene in which a senior surgeon is assisting his trainee to help her learn a new procedure. If he finds that the trainee is struggling to follow the steps and appears to be lost, the senior surgeon will ask the trainee to step back for a moment and, pausing during the procedure, will ask the trainee about her understanding of the procedure as it stands, current risks and the next step she envisages. In a way, the senior surgeon is trying to impart techniques of attaining situation awareness. This technique has been formally adopted as situation awareness global assessment technique (SAGAT) and has been studied in surgical specialties.[7] There are various other questionnaires available to assess general levels of situation awareness.

The recent innovation of Google Glass has been used to determine surgeons' attention while operating and may be useful to assess situation awareness. Google Glass is effectively a wearable computer with an optical head-mounted display. The heads-up display coupled with voice activation allows users to see and interact with information in a smartphone-like hands-free format.

SUMMARY

Situation awareness is remaining alert in order to maintain presence of mind during an operative procedure. In other words, it is a mental state in which you are fully aware of your actions and their effects and have a plan if you need to make changes in your actions. Maintaining situation awareness is a three-step process. It starts with information gathering about the existing situation, interpreting the information from other available sources, and using knowledge and experience to make sense of the information to take appropriate action. Stress and fatigue are important for their effect on situation awareness. The atmosphere in the operating room is bound to affect a team's situation awareness.

REFERENCES

1 Way L., Stewart L., Gantert W., Kingsway L., et al. Causes and prevention of laparoscopic bile duct injuries. *Ann Surg.* 2008; 78: 1109–14.
2 Dekker S., Hugh T. Laparoscopic bile duct injury: understanding the psychology and the heuristics of the error. *Aust N Z J Surg.* 2003; 237: 460–9.
3 Schwab S. *Cutting Remarks: insights and recollection of a surgeon.* Berkeley, California: Frog; 2006. p. 75.
4 Bromily M. Have you ever made a mistake? *RCOA Bulletin.* 2008; 48: 2242–5.
5 Simon D., Chabris C. Failure to detect changes to people during a real-world interaction. *Psychol Bull Rev.* 1998; 28: 1059–74.
6 Lockley S., Cronin J., Evans E., Cade B., et al. Effect of reducing interns' weekly hours on sleep and attentional failures. *New Engl J Med.* 2004; 351(18): 1829–37.
7 Hogan M., Pace D., Hapgood J., Boone D., Taylor R. Use of human patient simulation and the situation awareness global assessment technique in practical trauma skills assessment. *J Trauma.* 2006; 5: 1047–52.

CHAPTER 7

Primary stress management

Stress management is considered from two aspects, primary and secondary. Primary stress management is expected to reduce stress by modifying the inducing factors in the environment. Secondary stress management reduces the impact of stress by improving surgeons' ability to cope with these stressors. Thus the two aspects are complementary.

As seen earlier, the environment in which surgeons operate influences performance. Surgeons can control some of these environmental factors while others are beyond their control. Improving the operating room atmosphere can improve surgeon performance and reduce stress. Individually, environmental factors may not affect performance, but collectively they exert a significant influence.[1] All these factors interact with each other, thus, to manage stress, management of various factors needs to be considered.

NOISE

Noise is a harmful stressor. Ambient noise has effects on performance besides triggering negative physiological reactions like changes in cortisol and increased risk of cardiovascular disease. It decreases concentration and dexterity. In addition, noise in the form of communications can produce dangerous mental loading. The only form of noise that may be beneficial in the operating room is music, but that, too, appeals only to some surgeons, not to everyone. You may have experienced that in the operating room, on certain days, noise is produced by everyone and everywhere except from the point of activity, the operating table!

Many sources, including monitors, suction machines and conversations between individuals, contribute to the noise. During neurosurgical and orthopaedic procedures, the peak levels of noise can be as great as 100–120 dB.[2] Normal speech between individuals is measured at 60 dB. For speech to be clearly understood, it needs to be 10 dB above the ambient noise level. United Nations guidelines apply for workplaces including operating rooms. The recommended threshold of noise in the operating room is 55 dB.

The impact of a noise-reduction programme in an operation suite has been studied. After noise reduction was carried out, its impact on the rate of complications and on the surgeons' performance was assessed.[3] In 156 operations sound levels were measured before and after a noise-reduction programme. Surgical complications were recorded. The surgeons' biometric responses (cortisol, electro-dermal activity) and behavioural stress responses were measured and correlated with individual noise sensitivity.

Noise levels in the control group versus the interventional group were reduced by −3 ± 3 dB. The intervention significantly reduced non-operation-related noise. The incidence of postoperative complications was significantly lower in patients of the intervention group (n = 10/56 vs 20/58 control). Surgeons with above-average noise sensitivity experienced improved intra-team communication. The intervention reduced surgeons' pre- to postoperative rise in cortisol by 20%.

MUSIC

Some surgeons claim to perform better with music, but others fear it has a potentially disturbing influence. In his book *Music and Medicine*, Dr Desmond O'Shaughnessy reflected a strong disproval of music being played in the theatre … 'that amorphous effluvium of mixed sound sometimes even containing degraded threads of classical masterpieces, piped into operating theatres to distract, annoy or in some cases please the surgeon and other personnel there'.[4]

There is a perception that music has a strong influence on various psychological functions including emotion, verbal memory and even intelligence. Allen and Blascovich assessed the effect of music on surgeons performing challenging tasks in a research laboratory.[5] Fifty surgeons, who always listened to music during surgery, were asked to perform complex mental arithmetic tasks under three conditions: with no music, while music selected by the investigator was played and while the surgeon's chosen music was played. The surgeons were assessed for changes in cardiac responses, haemodynamic measures, electro-dermal autonomic responses, task speed, and accuracy.

Speed and accuracy of the task was highest when the surgeon selected the music played. Physiological measures reflecting stress were at a maximum in the no-music situation, followed by when experimenter-selected music was played. Stress was lowest when surgeon-selected music was played. No specific type of music was associated with any outcome measures. Thus it is not the type of music that affects the performance but the familiarity of the music to the performer. Taking it further, it is the listener's preference and not just familiarity that contribute to performance responses. The self-selected music may have caused the surgeons to feel better able to perform because of the past association of this specific music with positive performance. A particular type of music preferred by a surgeon may present a potential difficulty in that, while it may improve the performance and reduce the stress of the surgeon, it may have the opposite effects on the anaesthetist or other theatre staff. Their behaviour may negate the positive effect of music. It is important to note that it cannot be concluded that playing music is beneficial for surgeons who usually do not listen to it during surgery.

To examine whether listening to music during surgery influences performance of surgeons, researchers designed another study.[6] Surgeons who were not very experienced in simulated surgery performed a virtual procedure while listening to musical pieces of different emotional valence and intensity. It was expected that the surgeons' performance would improve under emotionally activating music. On the other hand, sedating musical pieces would have an opposite effect.

The researchers, however, did not find improvement in performance while surgeons were listening to activating music. In fact, they found the effect to be detrimental to the performance. The damaging effect of activating music was robust during the first trial and accompanied by a proportional increase in the stress response. However, this effect faded completely in the subsequent trials, demonstrating the ability of the brain to compensate for the disruptions. A previous study by Allen and Blascovich, which examined the influence of music on surgeons, showed different results,[5] attributed to the fact that surgeons in their study were music enthusiasts who had been listening to music while operating.

Thus it is difficult to see a beneficial effect of music on performance, at least among inexperienced surgeons. Music in the operating theatre might even have a distracting effect on a surgeon performing new tasks. This opinion has significance due to the fact that a novice surgeon does not have much influence on the choice of music played in operating room while learning a new procedure. A practical solution would be to switch off music during training procedures.

It is well known that multitasking capability diminishes as age advances. As age advances, the attention span diminishes and focus on a particular task requires full concentration despite increased experience in doing it. Dr Ravishankar Vedantam, a spinal surgeon from the USA, offered his personal experience: 'I used to listen to my selected music in my thirties and up to my mid-forties while operating on long spine cases lasting usually eight hours or so for a single case. However, I suddenly found music to be a distraction as I crossed the mid-forties age group.' Thus subjective personality changes may have something to do with the choice of listening to music or not during surgery. Overall, if music is played, it may be preferable for it to be played at a very low volume, blending with the ambient noise rather than being heard over and above the ambient noise. Besides, music in itself may add to the ambient noise and make verbal communication between staff members in the operating room difficult.

OPERATING ROOM TEMPERATURE

The temperature of an operating room is usually decided according to the patient's requirements balanced against the comfort of the operating room staff. Some anaesthetists like to turn up the temperature so that the patients remain normothermic. This may lessen surgeons' comfort. Although it is understandable to set the temperature according to the needs of the patient, one also needs to consider the comfort of the operating surgeon. A study on medical students in the UK found that 12% of respondents had suffered syncope in the operating room; of these, 79% reported hot temperature as a causative factor.[7] Moderate heat stress affects mental performance by reducing levels of alertness. Surgeons feel comfortable at an ambient temperature of 19–21°C. To compensate for the operating light, a temperature of 18°C has been advocated. Cooling vests like those worn by firefighters have been tried by surgeons and have been found very useful. Dr Vedantum adds his personal experience: 'I have used cooling vests (with ice cold water circulating through the vest) for almost eight or nine years for my long complex spine cases which I would do twice a week for fifty weeks in a year. I found that it dramatically reduced fatigue and helped maintain focus for the long days of surgery. Also, it would not alter the ambient room temperature, thereby allowing the anaesthesiologist to keep patient temperature at normothermic levels.'

POSTURE

Poor posture impairs psychomotor performance and worsens stress. Some surgical procedures require protracted standing and awkward body positions. In a procedure that lasts for many hours, sitting during part of the operation reduces body fatigue. A problem with sitting while operating is the shortage of leg space under the operating table. This is linked to a forward leaning posture that is a risk factor for back pain. Intermittent change in posture helps prevent prolonged and constant use of a particular set of muscles, thereby allowing for periods of relaxation for the muscle groups. For example, it may be beneficial to intermittently correct the posture of the spine to the normal vertical from the constant forward-bending posture associated with the performance of many surgical procedures. Operating in a seated position has benefits of better precision and stability and less energy consumption. Moreover, a saddle chair position offers a physiological lumbar spine position. Alternating between the standing and the supported-standing positions to avoid any prolonged specific posture is recommended.

The working height of the operating table has diverse effects on a specific muscle load. The load on a trapezium can go above advocated threshold in the standing position if the table is over 5 cm above the elbow level. The use of armrests in simulated laparoscopic surgery can reduce error rates and discomfort. Work-related pain could also be a factor in limiting or ending surgeons' careers due to musculoskeletal-related pain and loss of function. It therefore behoves every surgeon to be cognisant of the importance of ergonomics in the workplace.

OPERATING ROOM STAFF

The support from an experienced and familiar nursing staff reduces stress and improves coordination. The advantages of a dedicated team are known. In an ideal world the surgeon has to say little and the instruments should flow from the nurse's hand to the surgeon's without the surgeon asking for them. Experienced operating room staff carry out more anticipatory movements compared with less experienced ones. Reduced operating time and lower conversion rates are seen for laparoscopic procedures with a 'dedicated trained' operating team.

Higher complication rates can be anticipated when there is unplanned leave and regular staff are replaced by temporary staff. Higher complication rates may be attributed to the stress due to the individual being moved unexpectedly and the changed dynamics of the operating team. Unavoidably, operating staff may change unexpectedly but confirming that all team members have been introduced to one another can decrease stress associated with altered team dynamics.

The presence of inexperienced trainee surgeons has an effect on the dynamics of an operation. An experienced trainee who is familiar to the surgical team is able to improve the flow of surgery by anticipating the requirements and movements of the operating surgeon. On the other hand, trainee surgeons unfamiliar with the team take longer to perform operations, causing increased stress to complete the operations within time. A significant relationship is seen between time pressure and the incidence of operative errors. Time pressure is also a factor that negatively impacts on the trainee's experience.[8]

FATIGUE

The study of the effect of fatigue on surgical skills has shown cognitive performance to be more impaired than psychomotor skills. It is recommended that there should be greater emphasis in averting cognitive errors during times of fatigue.[9] In work situations where high performance has to be delivered over a prolonged time, short intermittent breaks are useful to reduce stress and errors. Air traffic controllers take breaks every 20 minutes. These kinds of practice are not applied during long operations. The image of the indefatigable surgeon has powerful sociocultural roots and many surgeons wish to maintain it that way.

Mountaineers consider the 'break schedule' as a key success factor for the historic first climb on Mount Everest. Traditional climbing involved a long break every 4 hours. In contrast, the successful expedition in 1953 climbed according to the so-called 'Sherpa scheme', which involved 50 minutes fast climbing followed by a mandatory break of 10 minutes. Enthused by this plan, Carsten Engelmann and colleagues in Germany decided to see if breaks during long operations lower the surgeon's stress response and improve performance.[10]

A randomised controlled trial was carried out in which complex operations were subjected to a break scheme consisting of 25-minute work periods followed by 5-minute unstructured breaks, during which the pneumoperitoneum was released (this was the intermittent pneumoperitoneum or IPP group). The control group consisted of operations performed without breaks, termed the CPP group (continuous pneumoperitoneum). Surgeons with experience of more than 300 laparoscopic procedures were monitored biometrically, by task measures and questionnaires. The primary endpoint was the hormonal stress response of the operating surgeon. The strain markers, cortisol, amylase (which served as surrogate parameter for adrenal activation), and testosterone were measured from the surgeon's saliva. Secondary endpoints included: continuous ECG, psychometric studies of concentration and performance, error rates, self-ratings of own performance and fatigue and musculoskeletal system (MSS) and ophthalmologic strain. The IPP and CPP operations were equally distributed among the surgeons.

The cortisol level of surgeons operating without breaks was 22% higher than of those operating with breaks. Also, continuous ECG found a significantly higher start–end variability in the CPP group. The performance test results in the CPP group had a decreased performance score and an increased error rate. In contrast, the IPP break scheme maintained the overall performance and error rates. The intergroup differences for performance were significant. The IPP error rate was threefold lower than the CPP error rate. The perceived impairment by fatigue was lower in the IPP group. Also, there was a decrease in surgeons' perceived stress. The preoperative values were identical between both groups, whereas postoperatively in the IPP group fatigue and perceived impairment by fatigue were significantly lower. The maximal perceived stress was also decreased, which can be explained by the fact that fatigue raises the workload and stress. There was a concern whether the benefits for the surgeon were at the cost of the patient. Surprisingly, the breaks did not prolong the operating time at all. Thus the IPP break scheme decreased the surgeon's stress hormones and the objective error–performance scores.

Dr Vedantum says, 'I would do intermittent stretching every couple of hours or even every twenty to thirty minutes (if using a microscope) during surgery to improve posture and reduce fatigue. I used my knowledge of anatomy to help me with what types of muscles needed stretching. Certain muscle groups act as storehouse of stress-related tension and they need to be stretched in particular.' Recent studies have shown that intraoperative targeted stretching micro breaks (TSMBs) may offer a practical and effective means to reduce surgeon pain and fatigue and enhance performance and mental focus without extending the operative time.[11] Sixty-six participants (69% men, 31% women; mean 47 years) completed 193 'non-TSMB' and 148 'TSMB' procedures. Forty-seven per cent of surgeons were concerned that musculoskeletal pain may shorten their career. TSMB improved surgeons' post-procedure pain scores in the neck, lower back, shoulders, upper back, wrists/hands, knees, and ankles. Operative duration did not differ. Improved pain scores with TSMB were statistically equivalent for laparoscopic and open procedures. Surgeons perceived improvements in physical performance (57%) and mental focus (38%); 87% of respondents planned to continue TSMB.

TIMING OF SURGERY

Shift work affects physiological systems. A drop in mental performance and decision-making capacity occurs from midnight till early morning. Alertness and performance have rhythmicity, with a maximum in the late afternoon and a minimum in the early morning. The risk of airline pilot error increases by 50% during the early morning. This is due to attention problems and fatigue. It is shown that protracted surgical procedures and reduced mental energy do impact surgeons' performance during different times of the day.[12]

SUMMARY

Primary stress management is expected to reduce stress by modifying the inducing factors in the environment. Adjusting operating room practices can reduce stressors like noise and interruptions. Retaining a consistent operating team, effective scheduling of procedures and sufficient time for a rest are some of the ways that are helpful for stress reduction. Deliberation needs to be given to posture and related ergonomic factors. Surgeons should scrutinise their operating room environment and recognise issues that they are able to change. By addressing these issues, operative results will improve but it will also enhance fulfilment with the workplace. The environmental changes cannot be solely left to the administrators and managers since, as responsible clinicians, surgeons have an obligation to their patients to improve the atmosphere in which they get operated.

REFERENCES

1 Wong S.W., Smith R., Crowe P. Optimising the operating theatre environment. *Aust N Z J Surg*. 2010; 80: 917–24.

2 West J., Busch-Vishniac I., King J., Levit N. Noise reduction in an operating room: a case study. *J Acoust Soc Am*. 2008; 123: 3677.

3 Engelmann C.R., Neis J.P., Kirschbaum C., Grote G., Ure B.M. A noise-reduction program in a pediatric operation theatre is associated with surgeon's benefits and a reduced rate of complications: a prospective controlled clinical trial. *Ann Surg*. 2014; 259(5): 1025–33.

4 O'Shaughnessy D. *Music and Medicine*. Brunswick, Victoria: Globe Press; 1984.

5 Allen K., Blascovich J. Effects of music on cardiovascular reactivity among surgeons. *JAMA*. 1994; 272: 882–4.

6 Miskovic D., Rosenthal R., Zingg U., Oertli D., et al. Randomized controlled trial investigating the effect of music on the virtual reality laparoscopic learning performance of novice surgeons. *Surg Endosc*. 2008; 22: 2416–20.

7 Jamjoom A.A.B., Nikkar-Esfahani A., Fitzgerald J.E.F. Operating theatre related syncope in medical students, a cross sectional study. *BMC Med Educ*. 2009; 9: 14.

8 Hutter M.M., Glasgow R.E., Mulvihill S.J. Does the participation of a surgical trainee adversely impact patient outcomes? A study of major pancreatic resections in California. *Surgery*. 2000;128: 286–92.

9 Gerdes J., Kahol K., Smith M., Leyba M.J., Ferrara JJ. The effect of fatigue on cognitive and psychomotor skills of trauma residents and attending surgeons. *Am J Surg*. 2008; 196: 813–20.

10 Engelmann C., Schneider M., Kirschbaum C., Grote G., et al. Effects of intraoperative breaks on mental and somatic operator fatigue: a randomized clinical trial. *Surg Endosc*. 2011; 25: 1245–50.

11 Park A.E., Zahiri H.R., Hallbeck M.S., Augenstein V., et al. Intraoperative 'micro breaks' with targeted stretching enhance surgeon physical function

and mental focus: a multicentre cohort study. *Ann Surg.* Feb 10, 2016 (Epub ahead of print).

12 Leff D., Aggarwal R., Rana M., Nakhjavani B., et al. Laparoscopic skills suffer on the first shift of sequential night shifts; program directors beware and residents prepare. *Ann Surg.* 2008; 247: 530–9.

CHAPTER 8

Secondary stress management

Being able to operate effectively under stress-inducing conditions is a hallmark of expertise, and developing such ability is important. To understand which factors play a part in achieving excellence in surgical performance, experienced surgeons from various specialties in Canada were once asked for their views and their preferred methods of preparing for surgical procedures. Of the three key factors, mental, technical and physical, mental preparation was regarded as the most important by 49% of surgeons. The technical and physical factors were considered to be important by only 41% and 10% of surgeons respectively. Thus, it was the appropriate mental preparation that made the biggest difference between desired and undesired surgical performance.[1]

We have seen the effect of stress on surgical performance; nevertheless, we don't know much about the relationship between stress-coping and surgical performance. Although there may be an acknowledgement that stress-coping responses play a role in performance, specific strategies for coping are not explicitly known or taught. A study was designed to assess the impact of stress-coping on surgical performance.[2] Surgeons were asked to perform a task on a simulator and while performing, they were exposed to very harsh critical comments to make them feel stressed. Before the participants performed the task their stress-coping style was identified by an assessment. The assessment focused on four specific coping styles: devaluation, distractions, controls over stressful reactions, and negative coping. The first three strategies (devaluation, distractions and control) are known to reduce stress while negative strategies make it worse. When people use devaluation strategy to cope with the stress they try to reduce the intensity or importance of stress by seeking self-assurance by saying things like, 'everything will turn out all right'. Some people using the same strategy will deny responsibility for stress creating situation by thinking 'it's not me who created this problem'. The strategy of distraction involves diverting the focus from stress-related situations or turning it to positive activities. Apart from these two common styles of copying, surgeons also employ 'control' strategy. The control may be either controlling the situation or it may be controlling the reactions. For controlling the situation you have to analyse the situation, plan actions, and act for control and problem solving. For controlling the reactions one has to encourage self-competence and ability to control. The negative coping style involves escapism, avoidance, guilt or over-dependence on others. To find out the correlation between coping and performance, the surgeons were assessed according to the time taken to complete the task, errors and economy of motion.

The results (Figure 8.1) showed a correlation between coping style and performance. Interestingly, for those who adopted a distraction strategy, the higher the score of the strategy, the worse was the performance. The coping strategy of distraction, however, is generally considered as a positive stress-coping strategy. Nevertheless, in the context of surgery, distractive thoughts appear to be counterproductive because the operator must concentrate on the task at hand. Thus in case of 'distraction', the correlation between coping and performance was negative. One of the helpful strategies was found to be 'self-control', which involved maintaining self-composure before addressing the stressful situation.

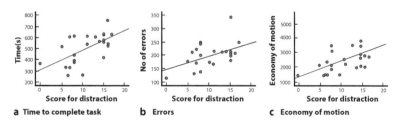

a Time to complete task   b Errors   c Economy of motion

Figure 8.1 Effect of coping on performance[2]

Another study assessed the impact of stress and coping strategies on performance of a simulated carotid endarterectomy (CEA) carried out by surgeons of diverse levels of experience.[3] The surgeons were grouped into two categories according to experience. 'Low Experience' surgeons had performed fewer than 12 CEAs while 'High Experience' surgeons had performed more than 12. The first scenario was a non-crisis procedure. In the second procedure, the patient suffered a series of crises: bradycardia on manipulation of the carotid body, stroke 3 minutes after clamp application, and stroke on shunt removal before final completion of the endarterectomy. Surgeons' stress was evaluated by questionnaire, interviews, observations, heart rate variability and salivary cortisol. Objective Structured Assessment of Technical Skill (OSATS) assessed surgical performance. The quality of the operative end product was assessed using End Product Assessment Rating Scale (EPA).

The effective coping strategies were significantly correlated to the surgeon's performance in both non-crisis and crisis procedures. During the non-crisis simulation, a high coping score and experience significantly enhanced performance. During the crisis simulation also, a significant beneficial effect of the interaction of high experience and low stress on all performance measures was found. Coping significantly enhanced non-technical skills as well. Thus stress and coping skills are important factors for the outcome of surgery when dealing with the challenges of complex procedures.

The researchers made two important observations (Figure 8.2). The first is that coping strategies enable the surgeons to improve their performance. And the second is that coping skills are independent of experience, implying that they do not develop automatically with surgical practice. However, experience was the greatest predictor of performance in both scenarios. During the non-crisis scenario, experience overruled the effect of stress; and during the crisis scenario, experienced surgeons with high stress levels did not show significant deterioration in performance. Surgeons' coping was unrelated to both experience and stress. While experience helps to counteract the unwanted stress responses, the specific coping strategy improves performance during challenging situations. Coping needs to be considered as a distinct skill that is a part of surgeons' competence. Stress and coping strategies are considerably correlated to the quality of surgical performance in addition to experience. Nevertheless, the fact that surgeons do not automatically acquire these strategies indicates that coping skills need to be nurtured in a deliberate manner.

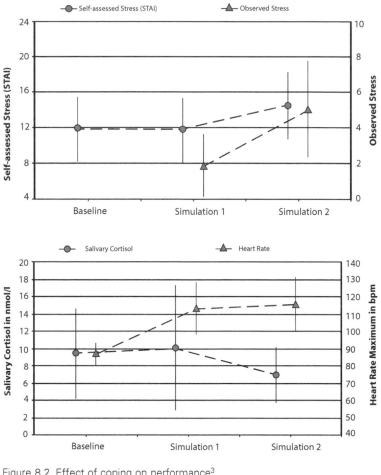

Figure 8.2 Effect of coping on performance[3]

If coping with stress is so important it becomes imperative to see if these coping strategies can be taught in a formal manner and also to find out if such training has any impact on performance. Whether training surgeons in copying strategies improves their performance was evaluated by Wetzel and her colleagues.[4]

The participants in the study were surgeons who were able to perform a carotid endarterectomy independently. Two groups were randomised to see the effects of stress management training on operative performance during a simulated carotid endarterectomy. In each group, eight participants were included and assessed during two crisis simulations. In the first simulated procedure, the patient underwent a surgical crisis: ischaemic symptoms 3 minutes after clamp application and stroke on shunt removal before final completion of the procedure. When the surgeon completed this task, the simulated patient recovered fully from the acute crisis. In the second simulated procedure the crisis reoccurred 5 minutes after shunt insertion and resulted in a loss of consciousness of the patient, indicating a stroke and the need for intubation. The intervention group received the stress management training after performing the first simulation. The control group received no training on stress management. Surgeons' stress levels were assessed using questionnaire, observations, heart rate variability and salivary cortisol. Surgical performance was assessed by Objective Structured Assessment of Technical Skill (OSATS); non-technical skills were assessed using Observational Teamwork Assessment for Surgery (OTAS); the quality of the operative end-product was assessed using End Product Assessment Rating Scale (EPA) and the surgical decision making (DM) was evaluated by observer's rating.

The intervention group showed a significantly lower level of mental strain than the control group. The intervention was beneficial to the use of coping strategies, surgeons' stress and their performance during a simulated surgical crisis. Physiological indicators of stress and psychological ratings of observed and self-assessed stress revealed a consistent pattern within each experimental group (Figure 8.3).

WHEN BAD THINGS HAPPEN TO GOOD SURGEONS

Despite surgeons' best intentions, patients occasionally suffer injury. The psychological toll of untoward incidents on a surgeon can be considerable, particularly if the harm is thought to be avoidable or causes serious consequences. For this reason, healthcare professionals are considered as the 'second victims' of adverse events.

A surgeon can be affected by serious untoward incidents. Even though the intense emotional reaction fades over time, certain cases remain in the memory for many years. Serious complications can make surgeons more conservative or risk-averse, which may not serve patients' interest.

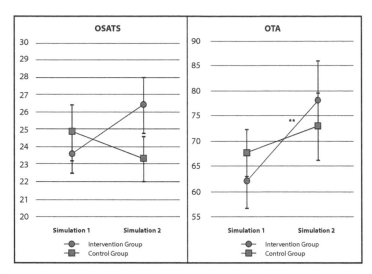

Figure 8.3 Improvement in surgical performance seen after training in coping with stress. Wetzel, C.M., George A., Hanna G.B., Athanasiou T., et al. Stress management training for surgeons: a randomized, controlled, intervention study. *Ann Surg.* 2011; 253(3): 488–94.

A sense of direct responsibility makes the surgical adverse event more personal than many other medical events.

Surgeons are considered to be more resilient than other specialists. However, there are differences in the nature of reactions. Some surgeons are more affected than others. Some are able to protect themselves from the distress like water off a duck's back while others completely fall to pieces. This variability can partly be attributed to experience. Personality also plays a role, but use of coping strategies is the critical factor. Experienced surgeons react less strongly and also possess more effective methods of dealing with those reactions. However, inexperienced surgeons are concerned about the repercussions of complications; therefore, the effect of an untoward incident on junior surgeons is especially significant.

In a study that discussed the impact of complications, all the participant surgeons were affected by a complication at some time in their careers.[5] Almost all surgeons disclosed that complications had psychological impacts on them, for a long time in some cases. The usual emotions were of guilt, anxiety, anger, crisis of confidence and worry about reputation. Some reported ongoing rumination and difficulty in concentrating. A feeling of personal responsibility and guilt was a recurrent theme. Younger surgeons felt anger towards their attending-consultant surgeon for inadequate supervision.

Over two-thirds of the surgeons said that grave complications had an influence on the way they practised. Although a complication is supposed to be a learning experience, many conceded that consequences of complications do not necessarily improve patient care; it may worsen it in some cases. The frequently observed impact was the inclination to become risk-averse. Preventable complications have a greater personal impact. Complications in elective surgery are more stressful than those in emergency operations where the expectations of death are higher.

Surgeons feel the existence of a blame culture aggravates the load of complications. For many, a blameless culture is a myth as institutions endorse a punitive approach to complications. Morbidity and mortality meetings are especially perceived in a negative light. These meetings are supposed to be important learning forums, but they seem to be dominated by blame. Rather than brainstorming, these meeting become 'blame-storming'. Everyone in the meeting is defensive and attempts to show themself in the best possible light. The blame is aimed at an individual instead of at procedures and style of decision making. Absence of institutional support and adverse comments from associates are barriers in effective coping as some surgeons consider help from colleagues as vital.

From a cognitive science perspective, coping mechanisms can be grouped under two types:

1. **Problem-focused coping** – this kind of coping is aimed at altering the relationship between the demands of the situation and the available resources. The common problem-focused coping strategies are: discussing the complications with colleagues to seek advice and to identify learning lessons and making efforts to update the necessary skills. For example, a senior surgeon would advise: 'Deconstruct the incident and replay it in your mind until you thoroughly evaluate it, how serious the complication was and how far you were personally responsible for it.'

2. **Emotion-focused coping** – this is aimed at handling the emotional consequences of the stressor. The common emotion-focused coping strategy is rationalising by putting what happened into perspective.

The stress gets reduced as you put things into perspective, since you remind yourself that complications happen no matter how good a surgeon you are, and should become part of your professional life. Other common emotion-focused coping strategies are talking openly to patients as a way of finding closure, and seeking reassurance from colleagues.

A possible consequence of surgeons' involvement in serious adverse events is the experience of traumatic stress. Anyone who has practised surgery knows that a major complication is a kind of 'gut-punch' for the surgeon. Few of us are fortunate enough to have had constructive mentoring to have developed appropriate coping mechanisms for dealing with such events.

Research was conducted to learn more about surgeons' stress in the aftermath of a surgical complication and how they coped.[6] Forty-seven general and vascular surgeons took part in the study. The surgeons were asked information about their complication such as how recent and severe the incident was. The impact of the incident was assessed with the Impact of Events (IES) scale. The stress score above 19 on this scale is considered to indicate severity of clinical concern. Surgeons' ways of coping were measured with the Brief-COPE inventory, which assesses the use of various coping strategies like self-distraction, active coping, denial, substance use, and use of emotional support.

The study revealed that one-third of the surgeons experienced traumatic stress of clinical concern during the first month after the incident. They also found that those who experienced stress used self-distraction as the method of coping. When someone tries to divert attention from a matter that is emotionally distressing, the person is said to be using self-distraction. Thus 'not thinking about the incident' or trying to use something else as a distraction is associated with higher possibility of post-traumatic stress. This is a known psychological phenomenon in which suppression of thoughts related to a traumatic incident is associated with greater post-traumatic stress disorder (PTSD) symptoms at a later stage. Self-distraction is seen when you say, 'I won't think about this today; I'll think about it some other time.' After hearing about an untoward incident a senior surgeon would say, 'Don't forget the event, think about it, talk about it, learn from it, decide what you can do to make sure it doesn't happen again, and then get back in the game.' Such an approach is useful. Surgeons who discuss complications with colleagues and use the experience as an opportunity for self-improvement experience fewer symptoms of post-traumatic stress disorder.

Many affected surgeons in the study experienced guilt, fear, and became hyper-vigilant in the aftermath of surgery that went wrong. These features are seen among individuals diagnosed with post-traumatic stress disorder.

PTSD is a syndrome associated with the experience of traumatic events involving three clusters of symptoms: (a) re-experiencing the event; (b) avoiding reminders of it; and (c) experiencing increased arousal.

The investigators tried to find out how some surgeons were able to cope without much difficulty. For those surgeons, discussing serious complications with peers or deconstructing the incidents to identify lessons helped. Another element was the extent to which surgeons felt themselves responsible for the problem. When surgeons feel that the problem occurred because of their own actions, they experience stronger emotional reactions.

A survey of 7900 surgeons found that those who had experienced a surgical error during the previous 3 months were more likely to have a lower quality of life and increased probability of burn-out and depression.[7] Thus the need for surgeons to have effective coping strategies is apparent. Surgeons cultivate these strategies independently, through observation and by trial and error. Stress management is not considered as a part of training or continuing professional development.

OVERVIEW OF SURGICAL COPING STRATEGIES[3]

Preventive coping – plans and checks to avoid stresses:

- planning the operation
- checking instruments
- team briefing.

Anticipatory coping – reducing inevitable stressors:

- awareness of stress
- knowing yourself: performance time and own limitations
- anticipating problems and backup planning

- early recognition
- accepting uncontrollable things and focusing on controllable aspect.

Proactive coping – enhancing personal resources:

- mental rehearsing
- practising technical skills
- broadening knowledge
- ensuring a good mental and physical condition
- scrubbing up process to 'get into a different mode' (calmness).

Intraoperative coping – control of self:

- stop and stand back technique facilitating physical relaxation
- calming down or remaining calm; reducing own stress responses
- checking to reassure one's own judgement
- self-talk
- focusing
- mental distancing techniques
- ergonomic adjustments.

Intraoperative coping – control of the situation:

- stop and stand back technique; gain time to think and to act
- reassessment and decision-making process
- intraoperative prioritising, planning and preparing
- team communication and leadership.

SPECIFIC COPING STRATEGIES

Here are some specific coping strategies used by surgeons. The investigators carried out individual interviews to explore surgeons' perception about coping strategies.[8] The coping strategies identified here are highly specific to intraoperative crisis management.

Early recognition of risks

The early detection of possible risk factors is vital for positive coping. Experienced surgeons identify inner indicators, such as distractive thoughts or clouded judgement, as signs of stress. On the other hand, inexperienced surgeons are unable to recognise stress or its effect on their functioning.

Stop and stand back

If unforeseen problems arise, surgeons may stop what they are doing and will buy some time; for example, by putting pressure on bleeding. By doing this they are mentally standing back and regaining self-control. They then would review the situation, make an appropriate decision and move to the next stage. It is better to avoid over-focusing on the problem and break the vicious cycle of anxiety and time pressure leading to confusion and inappropriate decisions.

Control of self

Appropriate exposure of the operating site, neatness of the field along with delicate tissue handling, gentle movements and relaxed communication reflect that the surgeon is in control. The flow of the procedure remains smooth, the communication in the operating room remains pertinent and the theatre staff is focused on every step of the procedure with responsive attentiveness. When needed they are able to act quickly but in a controlled manner. There is no hurriedness or panic. This requires not just competence but composure. A surgeon with a good composure helps create a calm environment for the other operating room staff. Creating this kind of atmosphere in the operating theatre requires a certain kind of attitude and ability that is possessed by a good surgeon. Those surgeons who do not develop these attributes experience disruptions in the progress of the procedure and the operating theatre becomes a potentially hazardous place. It predisposes the patient to a higher degree of risk of complications. Expert surgeons are aware of the importance of offering leadership to the team. In stressful conditions, they first confirm to themselves that they are in control. Key strategies are bodily relaxation methods, distancing and self-talk.

Relaxation

Bodily relaxation is a useful method to decrease stress instantly. Surgeons can use the stand-back time to use relaxation techniques like deep breathing or they may simply wait until their heart rate slows down.

Distancing

This is an alternative strategy for breaking the vicious cycle. Distancing from the stressor may be mental or physical. The surgeon may leave the procedure for a short period, thus distancing herself from the stressful atmosphere. With this method, she is able to think logically prior to resuming the procedure. Likewise, during a difficult operation she moves to a different area, later coming back to the challenging part. For some surgeons, standing back may not be a physical act but just a psychological action. They disregard previous decisions and start thinking 'with a clean slate' to reassess the situation.

Self-talk

Self-talk entails inner dialogue. Surgeons employ this approach to calm down, improve confidence and focus. They give self-advice about the decision making with rational comments like, 'I need to stay calm, I can deal with this.'

More information about self-talk is given in the next chapter (p. 109).

Controlling the situation

To manage a problematic situation, surgeons follow the stages of: reassessment; decision making; intraoperative planning; being a team leader for the team; and solving the problem.

Reassessment

The reassessment comprises (mentally) standing back, pinpointing the problems, underlining the source of the problem, and exchanging information with the team.

Decision making

The surgeon deliberates on different methods to solve the problem, concentrating on factors he is able to change and comparing probable results. Senior surgeons predict conceivable difficulties, prepare contingency plans, and prioritise before making an ultimate decision.

Intraoperative planning and preparing
When a strategy has been selected the surgeon gets ready for the subsequent steps. This includes making sure that all necessary equipment is available and guiding the team.

Team communication and leadership
Leadership and stress affect each other. It is the stressful situations that test the quality of leadership and the role of leadership is a stress factor in itself. In the operating theatre the leadership may belong solely to the surgeon or in a crisis can be shared with an anaesthetist or nursing staff. When the surgeon is a sole leader, not only does he have to maintain composure for himself but he is expected to support others.

Solving the problem
After a decision is made and the arrangements for the following step are complete, the surgeon puts the plan into practice to solve the problem. This in itself can have a comfortingly stress-reducing effect and lead to a positive feedback circle.

When there is a bad outcome some surgeons feel crushed by it. But others do not appear to be fazed; they just move on to the next cases. It's not that they don't suffer when something goes wrong or they don't see the pain in patients' or families' eyes. But they don't lose their composure, because that puts the next patient at risk. As has been said: you need to swallow the bad outcome and keep going – especially if you have made a mistake; the patient needs you to stay calm and fix it. At some point, when things have settled, you will need to sort out what happened. Did you apply the right procedure, did you execute it correctly and still lose the patient, did you misunderstand the problem or did you fumble in the middle of the procedure?

SUMMARY

Skills for coping with stress are vital for the surgical performance when managing the challenges of difficult procedures. Research has shown that development of these skills is independent of experience. Surgeons need to make deliberate attempts to develop coping skills. These skills involve preparation, emotional control, environmental control, aiming at the wider picture, retaining and reinstating order, and maintaining composure. Unhelpful stress-coping strategies are associated with poor performances. Coaching non-technical skills like stress management would help surgeons for the varied demands of the operating milieu.

REFERENCES

1 McDonald J., Orlick T., Letts M. Mental readiness in surgeons and its links to performance excellence in surgery. *J Pediatr Orthop.* 1995; 15: 691–7.

2 Hassan I., Weyers P., Maschuw K. Dick B., et al. Negative stress: coping strategies among novices in surgery correlate with poor virtual laparoscopic performance. *Br J Surg.* 2006; 93(12): 1554–9.

3 Wetzel C.M., Black S.A., Hanna G.B., Athanasiou T., et al. The effects of stress and coping on surgical performance during simulations. *Ann Surg.* 2010; 251(1): 171–6.

4 Wetzel, C.M., George A., Hanna G.B., Athanasiou T., et al. Stress management training for surgeons: a randomized, controlled, intervention study. *Ann Surg.* 2011; 253(3): 488–94.

5 Pinto A., Faiz O., Bricknell C., Vincent C. Surgical complications and their implications for surgeons' well-being. *Br J Surg.* 2013; 100(13): 1748–55.

6 Pinto A., Faiz O., Bricknell C., Vincent C. Acute traumatic stress among surgeons after major surgical complications. *Am J Surg.* 2014; 208: 642–7.

7 Shanafelt T.D., Balch C.M., Bechamps G., Russell T., et al. Burnout and medical errors among American surgeons. *Ann Surg.* 2010; 251(6): 995–1000.

8 Wetzel C.M., Kneebone R.L., Wolosynowych M., Nestel D., et al. The effects of stress on surgical performance. *Am J Surg.* 2006; 191: 5–10.

CHAPTER 9

Cognitive simulation – mental practice technique to reduce operative stress

WHY DEVELOPING SURGICAL SKILL CAN BE STRESSFUL

The changing patterns of healthcare delivery, greater accountability and shorter working hours have reduced training opportunities and experience. The mushrooming developments in technology have pervaded the orbit of surgery profoundly. These new techniques require the psychomotor skills of a nature not previously encountered. While minimally invasive surgery is a big boon to the patient, it is more demanding on the surgeon. Surgeons who had been practising before the endoscopic era had to acquire new skills for performing these new procedures to stay updated. Similarly, microsurgery has magnified and widened the choices of surgical treatments, as, lately, has robotics. Each advance in surgical technology has raised a distinctive interface between the operating surgeon and the patient's anatomy. The introduction of a new technique is followed by waves of learning curves, since new modalities change the dimensions of interface between the surgeon and the patient. This process can be stressful since the operating theatre does not make for an environment conducive to acquiring new skills of this nature. In fact, a significantly reduced potential for learning in the theatre environment is what an inexperienced surgeon is likely to find. A surgeon whose skills are limited and who is not well versed in the operating team dynamics is likely to feel very stressed.

While it's true that an operating theatre is far from ideal for getting to grips with newfound skills, it's also a fact that ways of training outside the operating theatre are not very conducive either. Being two-dimensional and devoid of the physical interaction, books or DVDs are not suitable alternatives. This is where cadavers, live animals or bench models offer a viable option. Each of these options has its benefits as well as limitations.[1]

Cadavers provide a correct anatomic representation but the tissue characteristics may not be as representative as on a living patient. Besides, cadaver training is costly, entails only a one-time use for a specific procedure and is in limited supply. Live animals are an option that ensures an appropriate tissue texture but animal care is expensive. Along with the restrictions of one-time use and an anatomy not entirely representative of humans, using animals does not always justify its worth. Animal welfare laws that vary from country to country, restricting such procedures, are also an inhibiting factor. Subsequently, dry laboratory models have become more popular. However, the general impression about the dry models is that they sacrifice fidelity for safety, availability, portability and reduced costs.

Against this background, upgraded computer technology opened the door to more advanced and higher-fidelity simulators. With the ability of computers to create various scenarios, simulation has evolved from its primitive mannequin stage. Since simulators are potentially available round the clock, it is possible for training schedules to be flexible enough to allow for other commitments and to be incorporated into other programmes. A particularly intricate skill may be rehearsed many times over, till such time that the surgeon has overcome the problematic issues before operating on a patient. Simulators are known to facilitate adequate training for various other high-risk tasks where opportunity is limited by danger or impracticality. Just as flight simulators let airline pilots be comprehensively instructed without endangering the lives of passengers, surgical simulators enable the acquisition of skills without posing a risk to the patient. Simulators also eliminate the risks of communicable disease to the surgeon imparted through sharp injury. In a nutshell, *a simulator has the potential to save patients from trainees – and trainees from patients!*[2]

Despite the benefits, the incorporation of simulation-based teaching in surgery has remained limited. Such training is typically confined to simulation centres, restricting their availability. Being more expensive than the low-fidelity variety, the use of high-fidelity models is not as widespread. Additionally, a closer scrutiny of simulation underlines the point that although methods vary, everything still depends on the physical rehearsal of the surgical tasks. It is obvious that practice is crucial in gaining expertise in surgical skills. Nevertheless, physical practice for multiple sessions at a simulation centre is an expensive proposition. It is also very time consuming and difficult to maintain over a period of time. Moreover, keeping to the recommended practice regimen is no guarantee of a surgeon's progress in skills.

The transferability of skills from a simulator is an important criterion in considering the benefits of simulators. Transferability reflects that skills acquired in one setting can be applied successfully in a different setting. The significant endorsement for simulators will be that their use results in improved performance in the operating theatre. The transferability of skills from simulators has been assessed in various studies – and some of the results are far from encouraging.

A study attempted to discover if practising on a simulator did translate into actual surgical performance – and the conclusion was not in favour of simulators.[3] Earlier research showed that the use of simulators could familiarise surgeons with procedures but was mostly confined to basic skills. Moreover, invalid tools were used to assess the skills transfer. The studies that showed the transfer of skills involving diverse tasks with the same simulator, however, showed no evidence that it improved performance in actual surgery.[4]

A study was carried out to evaluate the stress levels of surgeons during the transition from the simulator to the operating room, and the impact of the change in setting on the performance.[5] Surgeons were randomly divided into intervention and control groups. After the training group attained competence in laparoscopic suturing, both groups were tested on a live porcine, laparoscopic Nissen fundoplication model. Their performance was judged by means of objective scores. Stress levels were monitored by recording beat-to-beat heart rate (BBHR) variability; at baseline, after reaching competency (for training group only) and in the operating theatre. It was noted that baseline simulator performance and heart rate variability were similar for both groups. After attaining simulator competency, the trained group showed a reduction in performance in the operating theatre and a rise in beat-to-beat heart rate. A similar but lower increase in beat-to-beat heart rate was seen in the control group compared to the study group. The investigators concluded that the increased beat-to-beat heart rate observed in the operating theatre reflected stress and performance anxiety which explained the incomplete transfer of simulator-acquired skill. This finding was similar to that of other studies which demonstrated that surgeons who achieved expert level performance on simulators did not perform at the same level in the operating room.

Aviation has long used simulation with huge success for training. There are some resonances between the flight deck and the operating theatre, especially in terms of team function and crisis management. Where these parallels break down, however, is in the dexterity, which is central to the work of a surgeon. Even in an emergency, an airline pilot does not have to perform the complex manoeuvres that a surgeon has to make.[6] The other telling difference between surgery and aviation is that in surgery every patient is unique and different in their presentation or anatomy, while the variations in airliners are limited and pilots know the variations explicitly, before taking to the skies. For this and other reasons mentioned earlier, surgeons should not blindly adopt simulation technology from aviation despite some parallels between the two fields.

Rather than following aviators blindly, if we look around we may find that in many ways surgical performance is similar to the competitive sports performance. If we look closer, a surgeon's work is more like that of an athlete than that of a pilot. Both require intense concentration and complex fine and gross motor abilities. Both are routinely performed under considerable pressure and stress. Preparation for a surgical procedure, much like preparation for a sports performance, involves both cognitive and motivational aspects. Given these similarities, surgeons would benefit from adopting the techniques that have been proven to improve psychomotor performance in sports. No doubt, the aim for surgeons is not to win a competition, as it is for athletes, but rather to be competent and effecient in every procedure performed.

Thus it will be helpful to cross over disciplines and borrow the methodology of skill acquisition from sports. In sports, the complex and unusual movements are learned to a high degree of proficiency.[7] Similarly, a surgeon's subtle movements during operation are not part of day-to-day actions that are performed casually. So, the requirements of the unusual movements are akin to the ones sportspeople encounter. The perfecting of complex manoeuvring is the aim in surgery, one that is common to professional sport. Given such common ground, it seems logical to syndicate surgery and sports science in an interdisciplinary manner.

MENTAL PRACTICE IN SPORT

In competitive athletics winning or losing is a matter of just fractions of a second, where microscopic advantages or disadvantages determine the outcome. Given the huge investments in terms of time and energy and the magnitude of the consequences of winning, it is no surprise that athletes today are so desperate in the search for a winning edge in performance. At the elite level, physical abilities are often almost even and then it is the psychological edge that swings things in the winner's favour. Performance enhancement in sport is synonymous with doping-use of chemical substances. But one may not be aware that top athletes employ mental techniques more than any other technique to enhance the performance and reduce performance stress.[8]

The legendary golfer Jack Nicklaus says that hitting the ball to a certain place in a certain way is 90% mental. Nicklaus watched a self-produced colour movie in his mind's eye every time he prepared to hit a ball. In his own words,

> *I never hit a shot, not even in practice, without having a very sharp, in-focus picture of it in my head. First I 'see' the ball where I want it to finish, nice and white and sitting up high on the bright green grass. Then the scene quickly changes and I 'see' the ball going there: its path, trajectory and shape, even its behavior on landing. Then there is sort of a fade out and the next scene shows me making the kind of swing that will turn the images into reality.[9]*

World cup ski champion Steve Podborski describes how elite skiers use imagery and why it is such a valuable technique.

> *Another thing that gets you to the point where you are one of the elite is the ability to visualise not only the way it looks when you are going down, but how it feels ... the muscle tension that you actually go through when you make the turns, and to experience what attitude your body is in ... I feel what things will feel like and see everything run through my head. I have a moving picture with feelings and sensations. When I am doing these mental runs ... if I make a mistake, I will stop the picture and back it up. Then I run through it and usually get it right the second time. I run through the entire course like that.[10]*

Sports scientists are paying heed to the psychological phenomenon and how it works. They have delved into the kinds of mental practice athletes use to attain their goals, and the personal and situational factors that facilitate or obstruct the process. They have sought answers to whether mental practice enhances or hinders performance and how effective it is. The evidence affirms that mental practice does enhance the learning and performance of a skill as well as performance-related thinking. It helps athletes in routine situations as well as their responses in critical situations. By combining the information from research on athletes' experiences with mental practice, scientists have tabulated principles to use it effectively.

MENTAL PRACTICE IN SURGERY

In a study, experts in various surgical specialties were asked to share their views on achieving optimum preparation for a surgical performance. They revealed that a particular kind of mental practice was vital for mental readiness and stress reduction. The experts followed a regimen, a series of activities to induce a positive state of mental readiness before their surgery. A good plan spelled a clear sense of direction. A majority would anticipate the complications and also their solutions. 'What would I do if …?' is a pertinent question in devising plans to deal with the unknown. Verbalising potential complications, listing procedural steps and reviewing plans of action is a good formula for preventing stressful situations as well as dealing with them when they occur. Seven out of 10 surgeons surveyed made sure they had enough time to be mentally prepared for an impending surgery. A quiet place and time to reflect on, formulate a plan and being focused were their mantras.[11]

Another study was carried out to determine the effects of mental practice on surgeons' stress.[12] There have been studies proving the use of mental practice in improving performance of surgeons but this study was focused on the effect on stress. The hypothesis was that participants who mentally practise the procedure would be less stressed than those who do not, when they actually perform it. This was the first study to show that a short period of mental practice can attenuate the psychological, neuroendocrine and cardiovascular response to acute stress in surgeons.

A prospective, randomised controlled design included 20 inexperienced surgeons. After basic assessment, the surgeons were trained on a simulator. After an introductory training session, they were divided into either mental practice or control groups. Each participant performed five virtual-reality laparoscopic cholecystectomies. Then, the intervention group practised guided imagery with a facilitator using a mental practice 'script'. This script contained a sequence of procedural steps for the operation but, in addition, a set of detailed and vivid imagery cues designed to enrich participants' mental representation of the skill being learned. The intervention group carried out 30 minutes of mental practice prior to performing the procedure. The control group was involved in an unconnected activity. Stress was measured subjectively by the validated State-Trait Anxiety-Inventory (STAI) questionnaire and objectively by a continuous heart rate monitor and salivary cortisol. Both groups were asked to perform the procedure on the simulator and were monitored throughout the performance.

The results showed that, comparing the mental practice group with the control group, subjective stress (STAI) was less for the former. Also objective stress was considerably decreased for the mental practice group in terms of the physiological parameters. Substantial negative associations were found in relation to stress and imagery; that is, a higher imagery score was correlated to lower stress.

Given the fact that the subjective as well as objective results differed between the intervention and control groups, one can conclude that the mental practice intervention worked as a successful stress reduction approach. This inference echoes the conclusions in sports psychology that recommend that in addition to refining cognitive skills, mental practice helps in optimising psycho-physiological changes.[13] The possible mechanisms underlying mental practice may be acting as a kind of 'stress inoculation training'.

Many surgeons rehearse their operations in their 'mind's eye' ahead of time. Surgeons who perform complex surgery go over operation sequences by visualising the steps before the surgery – particularly when performing less familiar operations or when learning something new. It is important to clarify the difference between 'rehearsing the operation in the mind's eye' or 'visualising the operation' and the specific technique of mental practice that was used in this study. Mental practice in this context, or to be precise, cognitive simulation, is a method *'to create or recreate an experience of operative procedure in the mind using multiple sensory modalities'*.

This method contains three key points:

1. To create as well as recreate experiences in our minds. Thus, it is based on memory and creative imagination.
2. Absence of external stimuli – it is a sensory experience that occurs without any environmental props.
3. It is a multi-sensory experience. Thus it is not limited to visual sense but includes other senses like kinaesthetic, tactile, and verbal, etc.

Various terms are used to describe this type of mental process, like imagery, visualisation, going through the mind's eye and so on. But the most appropriate term to use is 'cognitive simulation'. Mental practice is a non-specific category of any form of concealed practice. Even 'thinking through an action' or 'talking one's self through the steps' are considered to be mental practice. However, in case of the cognitive simulation type of mental practice, multiple senses are employed in a particular manner. When cognitive simulation is applied in its true spirit, it has been shown to reduce intraoperative stress significantly. It is vital to understand the concept and techniques of cognitive simulation thoroughly for you to experience the benefits.

Imagine entering a dark room with torchlight. If you point the light beam in one direction, you see a coffee table. Turn the beam in another direction, and a TV set and sofa can be seen. What the narrow torch actually lights up are just parts of the objects, such as the legs of the table or parts of the TV set and sofa. It is the brain that fills in the unseen parts of the objects lit up by the torch and enables their identification as table, TV set and sofa. Now replace the narrow torch beam by a laser beam that is far narrower, just a little dot of light that provides minimal data to identify the objects. This would be an appropriate representation of how limited our senses are at receiving information from the outside world. Continuing the torch analogy, as you walk through the dark room, you may then become aware of subtle sounds, hints of light or the feel of the floor under your feet. In this way additional sensory gateways are opened up to increase the input of sensory information. Turning up the 'volume' of the relevant sensory perceptions is a key ingredient in improving a motor skill. Usually when we are standing, the focus is not necessarily on the distribution of pressure on the feet. By turning up the volume on tactile perception, the extra information may be used to adjust the balance between the feet. Turning up the volume on sensations of hands or finger movements will enable the skill of imagining movement kinaesthetically to improve. The impact of mental practice or cognitive simulation is in direct proportion to the development or fine-tuning of the information-gathering capacities of the senses. Just like a master painter who can distinguish between the subtlest of hues and shades, sensory images should be viewed with judicious discretion.

Cognitive simulation in this sense is like computer software, but a version designed for the surgeon's mind. It is a technique that programs the mind to respond in a certain manner. No physical props or outside stimuli are necessary, as it is an activity that can be engaged in while seated in a chair. Imagine a movement, and the experience in the mind's eye can be as vivid as it is when doing it for real. During intense and vivid imagery, the brain perceives and interprets images as being real. That is why cognitive simulation has immense potential and scope to be a boon and a blessing in the surgical arena, especially to prevent deterioration in performance due to stress.

Designing a personal simulator with mental practice

This kind of mental practice is a multifaceted technique. It is important to distinguish individual facets, although once you start applying, many need to be combined. This may be like beginning by putting things into separate boxes, only to mix and match the contents later in one box. If you are able to make this method work, it is like having a custom-designed personal simulator, for your exclusive use, available any time, which takes up no room and, above all, costs nothing!

SENSORY MODALITIES USED IN COGNITIVE SIMULATION

Among all the sources of sensory information in the surgical procedure, visual information is particularly important. Skilled surgeons accurately process volumes of visual sensory data while operating that guide their actions and regulate movements. The art of learning skills depends on how a surgeon perceives and applies relevant visual information. Good-quality visual information relies on two factors: vividness and controllability.

Vividness is the intrinsic characteristics of the image, its clarity and richness, and controllability is the manipulation, transformation and retention of the mental image. The vividness shows how imagery reflects the reality of the mental content. Besides clarity, vividness is also about sensory richness. It is a measure of the intensity of activity of the cognitive process underlying the imagery, and just how lifelike an image appears. Vivid imagery conjures up mental representations with the use of detailed sensory cues. Ideally, such mental simulation is very close to the actual experience of the movement itself, hence simultaneously increasing the exactness of imagery. In technical terms, vividness can be likened to resolution and picture quality of a TV: the higher the resolution, the better the image quality.

Controllability is image maintenance and modulation, the ease and accuracy with which an image is transformed or manipulated in the mind, and it is a key factor in the mental rotation of a perceptual stimulus. One has to be careful as images can be manipulated easily yet inadequately and the exactness of the imagery may thus be compromised.

People with high vividness and high control show the greatest improvement in performance with the application of imagery techniques. Those with low vividness and high control follow, while those with low vividness and low control come next and, last are those with high vividness and low control. In fact, the last category, high vividness and low control, may be detrimental to performance. Uncontrolled images lead to situations that may have negative consequences. It is therefore important for performers to learn to control their images. Skilled performers seem to have both better control and vividness than those less skilled.

The use of multiple senses ensures enriched and more effective images, but this is not always easy as most people prefer to use imagery in one or two senses only. It is estimated that approximately two-thirds of mental images are visual in nature. The ability to switch between imagery modalities is a skill usually seen among high-level performers. Of all the various modalities, the visual and kinaesthetic ones have received the most attention.

KINAESTHETIC SENSORY MODALITY

Kinaesthetic sensation refers to the sensory information from receptors about body part location and movement, and the movement of muscles, tendons and joints.[14] Kinaesthetic sensation is 'feeling the movement or the feel of the movement'. This involves creating the sensation of how it feels to perform an action, including the force and effort perceived during movement. It also involves the sense of position, balance, muscle tension, gravity and effort. For example, you may imagine how much muscle tension you would use to push your body into the air as you jump, or how much effort you need to stroke ahead through water when you are swimming.

With the five senses (sight, taste, smell, touch and hearing) we perceive the outside world and with proprioceptive senses we perceive pain and movement of internal organs. Proprioception is the third distinct sensory modality that provides information about our position and movement of our body. Proprioception is made up of two subsystems: kinaesthetic and vestibular systems. Although these two systems are separate, they are closely coordinated in their operation.

Imagery in different modalities elicits specific changes in the brain for the processing of information in the relevant modalities. In the visualisation of a task, the occipital region of the brain registers activity. In the movement imagery of the same task, the activity is in the frontal area and not the occipital cortex. Thus, visual imagery activates visual pathways and kinaesthetic imagery activates motor pathways. Visual and kinaesthetic imagery are distinct modalities, serve different purposes and provide different information in imagery. Both are important and their effectiveness depends on the purpose of imagery and the nature of the task being imagined.

Jacobson's experiments culminated in one that supports the relationship between the nature of imagery modality and the concomitant response. He attached bipolar electrodes to the bicep brachii muscle and a mono-polar electrode to the muscles of the ipsilateral eye. Amplitude measurements were made by a galvanometer. When subjects were instructed to visualise bending their right arm, an increased action potential occurred in the ocular muscles but was absent in the biceps. Conversely, when subjects were asked to imagine bending the right arm, muscular activity was observed in the biceps while ocular activity was absent.[15]

A close match between the sensory modality and the desired result will enhance the benefits of the imagery. A combination of visual and kinaesthetic imagery therefore is an effective approach.[16]

One study classified participants as:

1. High visual and high kinaesthetic
2. High visual and low kinaesthetic
3. Low visual and low kinaesthetic imagers.

The researchers' results of comparisons of how well the participants learned a skill using imagery showed that the first group, the high visual and high kinaesthetic imagers, were the best learners, while the low visual and low kinaesthetic imagers were at the opposite end.[17]

TACTILE MODALITY

Perceptions of touch are of particular importance to the operating surgeon. Just like vision, the human perceptual system has evolved to perceive information through the skin, and not by means of instruments that pass through surgical ports in the body wall of the patient. The skin on the fingertips is most sensitive and is of crucial importance to the surgeon. A surgeon is most acutely aware of the loss of this information when first operating with the endoscope. However, over time the perceptual system will adapt to the degradation of information. This adaptation process may vary between individuals.

A surgeon must be able to identify tissue properties and handle tissue in an appropriate manner. Haptic (touch) feedback could be used to detect small tissue surface irregularities, to regulate forces applied to the tissues to avoid damage, to manipulate delicate tissues, and for greater precision and accuracy in difficult procedures. We know the distinct disadvantage with image-guided surgical techniques is the considerable diminishing of haptic input for which a surgeon must compensate during the procedure. Lack of haptic feedback is the bane of robotic surgery as well. However, endoscopic instruments do provide some form of haptic feedback that a skilled surgeon can interpret into texture, shape, and consistency.

Tactile imagery is closely related to kinaesthetic imagery: in fact, the two can be, and are, combined under the tactile-kinaesthetic label. Distinguishing between the two is necessary since purely kinaesthetic imagery need not be elicited by touch but is a prerequisite for tactile imagery. The complex haptic perception process could be called active touch as opposed to a passive touch.[18] Brushing up against some object unintentionally is passive touch, while active touch is purposefully examining say, a gall bladder covered by connective tissue, or a pocketful of coins, and discerning size, shape, texture, border and mobility. The exterior of a gall bladder, though covered by connective tissue, can be sensed, and the values of coins in a pocket, though unseen, can be estimated. Haptic awareness forms a kind of visualisation, and the visceral cortex is one of the highest centres involved in the processing of tactile information.

SURGEONS' RELIANCE ON VISUAL AND TACTILE IMAGERY

Q You just opened the abdomen of a 62-year-old woman with gallstones on whom you are operating for presumed chronic cholecystitis. On exploring the abdomen, you feel a 4–5 cm vague mass in the head of the pancreas.

A I need to determine if it is rock hard or if it is just pancreatitis. There are stones in the gall bladder, so the mass could be a common duct stone. I would feel now for any enlarged nodes in the region, and then re-explore the abdomen to see if there are tiny metastases in the liver on the peritoneal surface or anywhere else.

Q You don't feel any metastases.

A I would do kocherisation of the duodenum to get my fingers underneath the mass, with my thumb on top and my fingers underneath the duodenum and behind the pancreas.

Q It is definitely a mass, but it is poorly defined.

A I see two choices for biopsy: insertion of a needle either directly into the pancreas or right through both walls of the duodenum from a lateral approach. I would try to avoid piercing the common duct. I would look at the common duct now and dissect the material over it. I would not take out the gall bladder until I knew the diameter of the common duct, because I may need the gall bladder to divert the biliary tract if the common duct is small.

Q The common duct looks to be about 1 cm in diameter, just on the borderline of being enlarged.

A I would try to get a cholangiogram in some way. I don't think I would want to get it through the cystic duct, because I would need to keep everything intact in case I need the gall bladder. Because I am sure now that there is a mass in the pancreas, although I'm still not sure if it is pancreatitis or not, I would stick a Travenol needle, one stick at a time, into the head of the pancreas – into the hardest part of the mass – to see if I can get a diagnosis. I would freeze each stick one at a time. I want to see if the results are negative. Having done that, I would try to do a cholangiogram through the gall bladder, realising that it is going to take a lot of dye to fill it. I would have to try to position things so that the gall bladder dye doesn't obscure the distal duct. I would stick a needle in the gall bladder in an area I probably would use for an anastomosis.

Q   The cholangiogram shows what seems to be a tumour at the distal duct. The frozen section shows an adenocarcinoma of the pancreas.

A   I know the cholangiogram is not 100% reliable. Now I would begin to ease my finger down along the posterior surface of the tumour, which I have now dissected out, to see if it is stuck to the portal vein. I would also isolate the superior mesenteric vein inferior to the pancreas and the superior mesenteric artery and begin to dissect out these areas. If they are free of tumour, I would now know that the tumour is probably resectable.

COMMENTS

In this think-aloud the surgeon attempts to present visual and tactile imagery while focusing on the details of the manipulations. The description focuses on what the organs are imagined to feel like ('rock hard' pancreas) and on actions that would be done in exploring (feeling for nodes) or operating (positioning things so that the gall bladder dye doesn't obscure the distal duct).

Although the surgeon is simply 'talking about organs' and does not seem to invoke any higher reasoning, a great deal of knowledge and thinking is still involved here. Strategies reflect sophisticated considerations and experience; for example, 'I would not take out the gall bladder until I knew the diameter of the common duct, because I may need the gall-bladder to divert the biliary tract if the common duct is small.'

VERBAL MODALITY

Verbal imagery or self-talk is conversation with oneself, covert or overt, speaking to oneself about the performance. In the context of performance, the frequency and content of self-talk create a mind-set within which the performer operates. Mind-sets created by thinking strategies influence the quality of performance, which is why developing the skills of 'intentional thinking' is advocated. The myriad mind-sets created by self-talk fall into polarised categories, such as self-defeating thoughts or self-enhancing thoughts: winners versus losers. It is easy to intuitively imagine the mind-sets that different thought patterns create within the performer. The ultimate objective of addressing the content of a performer's self-talk is to develop a process-oriented type of thinking.

What the performer thinks in relation to her performance can have a significant impact. The interplay between the performer's self-talk and imagery influences the triggering of specific motor programmes used in performance. This line of thought entails a vocabulary of trigger words used to facilitate concentration on the task at hand; the formation of appropriate images associated with performance; the proper mind-set for performance and the formation of motor programmes.

OLFACTORY MODALITY

The sense of smell is all-important for animals but much less so for humans. Still, olfactory images can be powerful because they have the most direct pathway to the brain of all sensory images. A smell can instantly conjure up as a flashback the distinct ambience of a place visited long ago. Smell attracts and repels humans like no other sensory stimulation. Though the olfactory sense may not be of practical significance in cognitive simulation, it is a barometer for the quality of imagery and ability. Some surgeons describing the imagery of an operation will mention the smell of burnt tissue after the (imaginary) use of cautery.

PERSPECTIVES OF COGNITIVE SIMULATION

The two different approaches in imagining a movement are visualisation with the 'interior view' or by producing a 'mental video'. The first type of imagery is called internal perspective and the second, external perspective. External perspective (Figure 9.1) means watching one's own body executing a skill as if watching oneself in a video recording, with someone videotaping an operation you are performing with the camera focused on you.

An internal perspective is creating a visual image, like looking through one's own eyes and simultaneously feeling the muscular contractions and sensations that occur during actual movement. The image is much more vivid as not only do you see everything happen – through your own eyes and not the camera eye – but you can also feel and touch the equipment with your hands, and there may even be the sound of machines during the operation.

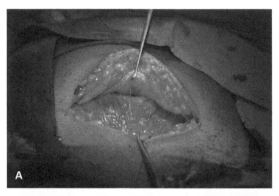

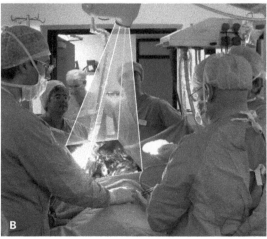

Figure 9.1 A Internal perspective (author's own image); B External perspective (reproduced with permission from Cuschieri A, Hanna G. *Essential Surgical Practice: higher surgical training in general surgery*, Fifth Edition. Boca Raton, FL: CRC Press; 2015).

An external perspective is most common in the initial stages of learning a skill, particularly if it is a closed task; that is, self-paced and predominantly under the control of the performer. An internal perspective is used to imagine well-learnt skills.

Both perspectives are extremely useful in skill development.

The benefits of external perspective are:

1. It is possible to move your perspective around and see the action from various positions (not available to the internal perspective) so you can analyse different aspects of the technique.
2. It can be used even if the task has not been executed before.
3. It may be primarily helpful when learning a new skill (especially by demonstration) or when you are trying to isolate and correct mistakes in skill execution.

The benefits of internal perspective are:

1. It provides a more realistic experience of the actual movement, providing identical perceptual information – you see the surroundings as if they were actually there and you feel the movements as if executing them.
2. It may offer more potential for performance benefits, because it has the potential to use all the senses and therefore should aid the transfer of training to actual performance.
3. It can be rehearsed by performers to practise procedure strategies, rehearse recognition of visual and kinaesthetic cues, identify and correct kinaesthetic movement problems and cope with debilitating performance anxiety.

Some say internal imagery is more effective than external imagery for enhancing performance, especially in procedures that have been performed repeatedly. Jacobson was the first to prove that internal imagery involves more muscle activity than external imagery.[15] Eye activity occurred in subjects thinking of performing a bicep curl (external imagery). In imagining a bicep curl (internal imagery), localised muscle activity took place. Internal imagery is also known to produce greater somatic arousal and less visual activity than external imagery.

The value of internal or external orientation could depend on the individual's level of experience with cognitive simulation. There are benefits to be gained from switching perspectives: just as visual and kinaesthetic imagery refer to different sources of information, internal and external imagery also refer to different sources of information and a first-person or third-person perspective.

TEMPORAL ASPECT OF COGNITIVE SIMULATION

Time is also a valid factor en route to successful imagery. The transit time for an imagined walk and (mental) arrival at a specific destination is remarkably similar to the actual time taken to physically walk that distance. The interest in imagery speed manipulation is of recent origin. Kosslyn in his renowned study used an image-scanning paradigm to prove that more time was required to scan longer distances mentally.[19] Similar temporal equivalence has been established through a large variety of motor tasks regarding motor imagery per se, proving that changing motor imagery speeds is sufficient to elicit changes in the timing of actual movement.[20] This conclusion can be used to improve the speed of actions. At times, even if actions become habitual and smooth, the performance remains slower than expected. In view of the imagery and real-time equivalence, faster imagery time would speed up the movements.

One can also use slow motion imagery for each component to help participants see each part clearly. This imagery technique can be particularly useful while learning a skill. Slow-motion replays of a task can give a clearer picture of its progression and can also be a boon in high-speed skills that are to be completed in a second or two. Important bodily cues or components such as a particular arm position can be easily identified and practised through slow-motion imagery.

Slow-motion imagery could prove difficult at first but does improve with practice. However, as the normal execution is at real speed, the maximum benefits cannot be transferred from practice to performance by overemphasising slow-motion imagery. It is best to conclude a session with normal-speed imagery so that the mental rehearsal speed matches actual performance, and hence maximises the transfer of practice.

POSITIONING FOR COGNITIVE SIMULATION

The recommendation is to adopt a relaxed position in the initial days of imagery training. Being at rest when using imagery means not reinforcing habitual patterns of movement. Being relaxed is conducive to being focused in imagery experience, thanks to reduced somatic tension and the elimination of distractions. A relaxed position sets the stage for the production of vivid images.

However, some people argue that relaxation could have a negative impact on performance as it inhibits the possible transfer effects of practice; the individual will not be relaxed during the actual performance so relaxed imagery practice may actually be detrimental to the impending performance. Thus, a pragmatic approach would be to adopt a relaxed posture only in the beginning of the imagery. Relaxation before imagery practice ensures it is more vivid and better controlled, which in turn makes it more effective. The aim is not to keep the subject totally relaxed throughout mental practice, but to use relaxation to induce vivid imagery.

As such, imagery can be practised in a variety of situations or positions such as sitting, walking or while waiting for the patient to be brought to the operating theatre. There is much to be gained by using imagery during other everyday moments; this also means a constructive use of unproductive time.

In some cases, bringing the body into a position similar to the task and moving slightly helps in the generation of a motor image. Imagery is generally performed without movement in the interest of improving performance, but there are advantages in performing imagery while moving slightly, or in positioning that relates to the target movement.

COGNITIVE SIMULATION SCRIPT

The content of the imagery is a crucial factor in its practice. Cognitive simulation is like installing a program into the human body as if into a computer drive. The outcome then will reflect the programming quality. If what is practised through imagery is incorrect, the eventual performance will in all likelihood be inadequate. Correct practice makes perfect while incorrect practice makes for imperfection. Careful planning of the content of imagery will maximise its effects in the effective acquisition of imagery skill. Ideally, surgeons could write their own imagery script to be used for a procedure.

For the maximum benefits from imagery the individual needs to be conversant with the procedure. To gain familiarity, imagery scripts must lay emphasis on underpinning the imagery representation of the skill. Such a script typically includes thorough directions on how to perform a procedure and also clues from diverse sensory modalities that enhance the experience. The aim is to facilitate a precise mental representation of the skill that is to be improved. Some of these are visual cues, kinaesthetic cues and cognitive cues; for example, task-relevant thoughts that go through the mind while performing the procedure. It is widely believed that movement-related kinaesthetic sensation plays a major role in imagery instructions. The kinaesthetic aspects of imagery, for instance, call for a focus on how the hands or fingers feel during movement or imagined movement to facilitate kinaesthetic sensations.

Some studies on imagery have shown conflicting results. With poorly reported instructions for imagery, the benefits of differing perspectives adopted during the process remain nebulous. Factors that could be responsible for this variability include the nature of the instructions and the variability of individuals in conducting imagery. Unclear or ambiguous imagery instructions may cause the content of the image to differ, significantly compromising the similarity with the physical task, and therefore the predicted development of the skill.

WRITING A COGNITIVE SIMULATION SCRIPT

Writing a procedure script can be seen as a three-step process:

Step one – core content: Outline the basic content of the procedure or situation to be imagined. Write it in the first person (I) if it is being used for yourself or the second person (you) if it is to be read to someone else. In describing how a skill is executed, ensure all components are included as well as the correct behaviour emphasised, especially if it is complex in nature.

Step two – the details and sensory stimuli: Use descriptors (adjectives) that add colour, detail and movement (e.g. the speed of the movement) to the original script components or events. Add movements or kinaesthetic feelings, body responses and emotional responses.

Step three – refining the script: You may want to rewrite components or actions into a paragraph that can be read easily and clearly. Reread it and try to imagine the event in all its sensory, action and emotional details. Do you feel as if you are actually executing the skill or experiencing the event? If not, re-examine the description to see if it accurately reflects the sensations associated with this action.

Cognitive simulation script

Here is an example of a cognitive simulation script prepared by an experienced orthopaedic surgeon, Duncan Learmonth, UK. It contains the tasks of the knee arthroscopy with sensory cues. These sensory cues are graphic coded – you are expected to do what each of the graphics represents:

👁 Call up a detailed picture in your mind. (Visual modality)

💬 Experience what you might say. (Verbal modality)

🔊 Experience what you might hear. (Auditory modality)

✋ Feel the action. (Kinaesthetic modality)

🖐 Feel the touch. (Tactile modality)

Positioning and preparation

✋ Imagine entering the theatre.

🖐 Transfer the patient and position on the operating table.

👁 Check tourniquet properly applied and as proximal as possible. Check position of leg post.

🖐 Scrubbing up, maintaining sterility with gowning up.

👁 Check position of stacker system and stool with wheels. Check tourniquet inflated.

💬 Verbalise patient's name and procedure.

💬 🔊 Hear and respond to Word Health Organization (WHO) check.

💬 Ask operating room staff to hold leg up by heel.

🖐 Prep the knee thoroughly. Clean thigh and calf. Apply drapes.

🖐 ✋ Position stool and sit. Flex knee to 90 degrees with foot in lap. Position foot pedals.

The operation

Infiltration with LA and adrenaline

👁 Look at knee; visualise what is medial, what is lateral.

📟👁 See and feel the lateral joint line corner of patella tendon and patella. Infiltrate with LA and adrenaline.

📟👁 See and feel the medial joint line. Infiltrate with LA and adrenaline along the joint line.

📟👁 See and feel the superior lateral portal. Three fingers superior to patella and midway on thigh anterior to posterior. Infiltrate with LA and adrenaline.

Making portals

📟 Feel lateral joint line, visualise the incision site corner of patella tendon lateral inferior border of patella.

✋ Take scalpel and make lateral incision at above location. Feel knife blade through skin, fat and then some resistance through the capsule. Aim knife to centre of the notch. Make cruciate incision in capsule.

Insertion of scope

✋ Hold scope sheath and obturator combination in dominant hand and push through lateral portal in direction of notch.

📟 Feel the tip of the obturator, push through the capsule and touch the notch area.

✋ Move the knee from flexion to extension, slightly withdraw the obturator and then advance the obturator underneath the patella and fully into the suprapatella pouch as the knee moves into full extension.

📟 Remove obturator from sheath and insert scope.

📟 Connect fluid tubing to the inflow port on the scope.

🗨 Ask scrub nurse to check that white balance has been carried out, shaver and ablator connected.

Diagnostic arthroscopy

Turn fluid on.

See fluid distend suprapatella pouch. See air bubbles.

Make stab incision in superolateral area and insert Wolf cannula for drainage cannula. Drain knee of air bubbles and debris until view is clear.

Connect drainage tubing to Wolf cannula.

Look at the undersurface of the patella by placing the light lead in line with the cable of the camera head.

Slowly withdraw the scope.

The upper pole of patella comes in view. Check the articular cartilage surface: medial, central and lateral.

Continue to slowly withdraw the scope.

View the patella from superior to inferior pole with the scope under the middle of the patella.

Move the light lead to the horizontal position on scope's medial side.

Move scope medial and lateral in sweeping motion.

View the femoral trochlea. Check the articular cartilage. Trochlea maybe obscured by fat pad.

Move scope to lateral gutter and move light lead to top vertical position. Move the scope down to the joint line.

View down to jointline; look for loose bodies and synovitis.

Move scope back to femoral trochlea and then move scope into medial gutter position light lead vertically. Move scope down to medial joint line.

View down the medial gutter to the medial jont line. Look for loose bodies and synovitis.

Place the scope in the medial gutter. Hold the scope in this position.

Hold the leg by the heel with the leg straight and abduct the leg. Move your body between the operating table and the leg.

(🖐)(💉) Allow the leg to be stabilised between the post and the side of your body and apply valgus stress to the knee.

🖐(💉) With this leg in this stable position,

🖐(👁) move the scope into the medial compartment and slightly flex the knee and increase the valgus stress on the knee.

🖐 Place the light lead medially.

(👁) Visualise the posterior horn of the medial meniscus.

(👁) Look for a meniscal tear. If shape of meniscus is not normal, think of a hidden flap either in the posterior compartment or flipped under the body of the meniscus.

🖐 The diagnostic arthroscopy is now completed. The tourniquet is released, the knee irrigated and the portal wounds closed.

🖐(💉) Local anaesthetic is injected into the joint.

APPLICATIONS OF COGNITIVE SIMULATIONS FOR STRESS REDUCTION

Cognitive simulation has immense potential to be a boon and a blessing in the surgical arena. However, its value reflects how well it is understood and whether the technique is applied correctly. Its application is influenced by a number of variables, primarily the various goals the surgeon seeks to achieve through its use to enhance performance.

 Cognitive simulation has a wide range of applications in reducing stress while operating.

Acquiring skills

Surgical skill acquisition taken place in three stages, namely cognitive, associative and automatic. The cognitive stage involves working out actions that are usually implicit, to make them explicit. For example, it will help an inexperienced trainee to focus on just what is involved in the insertion of a trocar for a laparoscopic procedure. A trainee with more experience could review the various stages of such an operation, which he has previously only observed. An experienced surgeon meanwhile may rehearse the variations that could occur in the course of a more complicated presentation.

Cognitive simulation can be applied in all three stages of skill acquisition. It can be applied to a review of anatomy as it can help surgeons become oriented in complex anatomic areas. Accurate mental representations of structures in the vicinity of a dissection will ensure more efficient planning of manoeuvres. Trainees should be encouraged to form mental images as they observe procedures. Such images can consist of visible anatomy but also, and perhaps more importantly, of structures not yet exposed. As learning evolves to the stage of automation, cognitive simulation assumes a form of risk management. To elaborate, while a novice will be concerned with what to do next to complete a procedure, an expert surgeon only thinks about key steps of operations, even in the case of rare or complex operations.

Shortening the learning curve

It is important to recognise cognitive approaches to minimise the learning curve of surgical procedures. Too much emphasis is given to the volume of operative experience, rather than the quality of learning experience. Of what use are logbook entries of operations unless active learning processes complement them?[21] Indeed, methods of teaching surgical skills outside operating theatres are interesting, but their nature and the extent of their usefulness is not well known. In particular, there is a need for programmes following workshops to maximise skill retention and advancement. This can be fulfilled by cognitive simulation.

Maintaining the level of skill

Could cognitive simulation be used to perfect an existing skill? In this latter stage, it can be assumed that a clear template of the skill exists. The surgeon already knows how to execute the appropriate movement: the goal now is to increase the chances of perfectly executed movements whenever required.

Top-level sportspeople are known to use imagery to enhance their skills. For elite performers, the positive effect of imagery may relate to maximising the transfer of skills from experience to actual performance. Cognitive simulation may enhance a novice's skills by reinforcing a template of the task. At higher skill levels, it serves to enhance efficiency by strengthening the cognitive template. It also maximises the cognitive focus of the performer by improving concentration and reducing skill-disruptive levels of arousal. At expert levels of performance, the skill level may well be close to a ceiling effect, leaving little room for actual skill enhancement. Thus, the value of cognitive simulation for top-level performers may mostly lie in ensuring the transfer of skills to actual performance.

Examining performance problems

Cognitive simulation goes well beyond mere intellectual activity, the thinking about or attempting to recall an event. When the action scene is 'switched on', the details of the event are activated. Unlike a movie experience, the performer is not just sitting and watching but is actually experiencing the event. Cognitive simulation becomes a type of instant replay, enabling the performer to closely attend to what was happening. An application of this phenomenon is for the re-experiencing of a procedure that has gone wrong.

Surgeons usually have their own take on what transpired during difficult procedures, and some will be adamant about the accuracy of their recall, until shown a video replay.

Surgeons can scrutinise their below-par performances by means of cognitive simulation to determine and detect the potentially confounding factor. They can then focus on why the error occurred and what could have been done to prevent it. It is important for them then to revisualise the experience and substitute the correct response.

Performance-related use

Cognitive simulation can also find an application in preparations for actual surgical procedure. Getting to grips with the technique in a laboratory or on a simulator both fail to replicate the conditions of the operating theatre environment. This is where the capacity of cognitive simulation to conjure up real-life conditions proves to be of immense value.

The skills a surgeon acquires have practical implications, which mean they are to be performed in real time and in the real world. Practice is the preparation, and performance is the execution of what has been learned. A conscious focus is necessary for a beginner to improve a skill that is being acquired and practised. That being said, an ideal performance should be effortless, as the technique of what is being executed is ingrained and stored in the subconscious. It is this unconscious competence that plays out in real-world performance. It is possible to have control over the environment during practice, but a performance entails an element of stress, known as performance anxiety. Physiological stress is an integral part of any performance. It is when it assumes pathological proportions that it casts a negative shadow over skills and thereby over the outcome as well. There is no way to rein in or harness all the stress-inducing factors, but it is possible to reduce the undesirable impact they have on performance.

- **Pre-performance cognitive simulation:** The mental practice of a well-learned skill prior to an actual performance can influence the motivational system (e.g. to reduce anxiety or boost self-confidence). It could even be used to modify the cognitive system by consolidating the accurate sequencing of a complex series of movements.

- **Cognitive simulation during performance:** The imagery experience can no longer decouple from the action itself. Rather, imagery is placed along a continuum extending from the overt movement to its mental representation. This has led to the belief that imagery could be performed not only before, or after, but also during the physical execution of the movement. It is beneficial for both concentration and the anticipation of forthcoming events. Imagery, therefore, is akin to action simulation, which involves the representation of the future and prospective judgements.

- **Post-performance cognitive simulation:** To review the negative as well as positive aspects of the performance. The performer should be aware of what contributed to a positive performance. Distinguishing the factors that lead to success and developing strategies to enhance performance in similar situations in the future will improve consistency. Imagery can be used to review previous peak performances, which will reinforce the belief that it can be done again, boosting confidence effectively.

Becoming familiar with unknown situations

At the elite levels of international sporting competitions, the venues are photographed for the benefit of competing athletes, who study photographs of the pools, fields, arenas, dressing rooms and even warm-up areas so that they can create effective images and see themselves performing there. This helps in familiarisation with the environment before the actual competition.

Similarly, surgeons too can visualise unfamiliar operating theatres where they will be performing in the future. A surgeon who has been using cognitive simulation visits five different hospitals a week to perform operations. He has successfully started using cognitive simulation to help him feel at ease in and adjust to the different operating theatre environments.

Practising psychological skills

Athletes who can handle stress remain focused in spite of distractions and confident in the face of setbacks; they are the ones who excel. Occasionally surgeons may get frustrated by something that has happened before they arrive at the operation suite or get distracted by theatre conditions or they may fret over the anaesthetist's actions. All this can and does influence whether a surgical procedure will go ahead as smoothly as it should. A surgeon's job throws up problems constantly, both in the theatre and outside. Strategies are needed to cope with stressful situations, which are acquired through experience or by trial and error rather than via formal training. Cognitive simulation can accelerate and enhance the strategy-evolving process by systematically developing appropriate techniques for specific occasions. The concept of mental skills training is new to surgery, but the importance of being able to cope with adversity has been known for a long time. Surgery involves performing both physically as well as mentally. Peak performance remains an unattainable dream unless a surgeon develops the psychological qualities marked by the three Cs: *commitment, concentration and confidence.*

Commitment

Cognitive simulation has both a cognitive as well as a motivational function. Motivational imagery focuses on end results or goals to be achieved. Commitment involves developing motivational skills that encourage the performer to improve, even when immediate progress is not apparent. Without commitment, no challenging long-term goals can be achieved and performance enhancement will remain a dream.

Perhaps one of the intriguing aspects of cognitive simulation is how it can focus a surgeon's resources towards the attainment of a specific goal. Specific goal imagery is like a self-fulfilling prophecy. The internal images that surgeons have of themselves tend to influence overt behaviour. Performers who see themselves 'choking' under pressure will most likely do just that in a critical situation. However, performers with successful images of themselves will often emerge as successful despite trouble and pressure. The formulation of a goal image activates the mind towards attaining it. Without a specific goal image, the mind cannot focus on the resources needed to attain it.

Concentration

Concentration entails maintaining undiluted focus during performance, devoting attention to important task cues and responding quickly and correctly to any circumstance. Surgeons need to switch their attention during procedures to both broad and narrow foci, externally to environmental cues or internally to strategies. As with other skills, practice in attending to various cues during training is essential to ensure that the focus is maintained during critical situations.

Cognitive simulation can be used to rehearse the focusing and refocusing of plans during a stressful procedure. In the case of a mistake or an unexpected turn of events, one can return to the proper task cues for appropriate implementation.

Confidence

In some aspects, confidence is a by-product of preparation for surgery. Self-confidence comes into being with the belief in success and in one's own competence. Confidence is enhanced by past success in a procedure and also by imagining a successful completion. Those who believe in their mind that they can succeed have greater chances of succeeding in the actual procedure. Replaying successful performances in your imagination will bring about positivity in your ability to succeed. If observing another surgeon demonstrating the proper execution of a skill can enhance self-confidence, imagine what the imagery of you succeeding in the same skill could do!

Sports science suggests that coping imagery has a greater effect on self-confidence than mastery images. Mastery images involve imagining the perfect execution of a skill, while coping images involve imagining the overcoming of an obstacle or difficulty during performance and eventual success. The latter being closer to reality, coping images should be used first, and the mastery images in conclusion, to conjure up a perfect performance.

COGNITIVE SIMULATION TRAINING

To derive maximum benefits from cognitive simulation, the approach must be effective. An inappropriate application may lead to the conclusion that it does not work. An image that flickers like a candle in the wind is far less effective than one that is steady and long lasting. The ability to transform an image is an invaluable asset in getting to the goals of movement. Here again, the ability to manipulate images is indispensable. Practice will ensure a familiarity with the many approaches in the learning of the most effective and constructive use of cognitive simulation.

One may think of 4 Rs in relation to cognitive simulation training. They stand for relaxation, realism, regularity and reinforcement. A relaxed state is conducive to producing vivid images. Realism means conjuring up imagery as real as actually executing the skill. Clarity, vividness and control are key factors in invoking the most realistic imagery. Practice also must be regular for optimum benefits. Reinforcement implies using visual or kinaesthetic aids to enhance the quality and control of imagery.

I have observed that expert surgeons employ the principles of these techniques, although they may not be aware of the name 'cognitive simulation'. As with many other skills, they developed these skills on a trial and error basis. With the new understanding and realisation of potential benefits to stress reduction, it is important to develop this skill in a deliberate manner. Once I observed a relatively young surgeon handling a critical situation very well. During the debriefing session, he was applauded for the way he handled the stressful situation and was asked: 'Is handling stress in your genes?' He answered, 'No, it is because I practised in my mind many times with different variations, in stressful situations. I never think of failing: I think of all the past times I have succeeded in my mind.' The cognitive stimulation immunises you to the stressful situation because it reduces anxiety, avoids distraction, guides behaviour and helps you focus on what helps you.

SUMMARY

Cognitive simulation can be used as a secondary stress management strategy that could help prepare surgeons to perform optimally under highly stressful conditions. Apart from its undoubted efficacy in this regard, cognitive simulation has the additional appeal of being inexpensive and easy to run — features that make it an attractive option in the current economic climate. Incorporation of cognitive simulation into surgical practice will assist in reducing stress enduringly, and in minimising the chronic effects of stress, including cardiovascular risk, on surgeons. Cognitive simulation has immense potential to be a boon and a blessing in the surgical arena. However, it is only as valuable as its proper application.

REFERENCES

1 Wong J.A., Matsumoto E.D. Primer: cognitive motor learning for teaching surgical skill: how are surgical skills taught and assessed? *Nature Rev Urol.* 2008; 5: 47.

2 Cosman P.H., Cregan P.C., Martin C.J., Cartmill J.A. Virtual reality simulators: current status in acquisition and assessment of surgical skills. *Aust N Z J Surg.* 2002; 72(1): 30–4.

3 Kavic S.M. Training and working in high-stakes environments: lessons learned and problems shared by aviators and surgeons. Perspective of a surgeon educator/trainer. *Surg Innov.* 2009; 16(2): 187–95.

4 Strom P., Kjellin A., Hedman L., Wredmark T., Fellander-Tsai L. Training in tasks with different visual-spatial components does not improve virtual arthroscopy performance. *Surg Endosc.* 2004; 18(1): 115–20.

5 Prabhu A., Smith W., Yurko Y., Acker C., Stefanidis D. Increased stress levels may explain the incomplete transfer of simulator-acquired skill to the operating room. *Surgery.* 2010; 147(5): 640–5.

6 Kneebone, R. Practice, rehearsal and performance: an approach for simulation-based surgical and procedure training. *JAMA.* 2009; 302(12): 1336–7.

7 Orlick T., Partington J. Mental links to excellence. *Sports Psychol.* 1988; 2: 105–30.

8 Lloyd P.J., Foster S.L. Creating healthy, high-performance workplaces: strategies from health and sports psychology. *Consult Psychol J.* 2006; 58(1): 23–39.

9 Nicklaus J. *Golf My Way.* New York: Simon and Schuster; 1974. p. 79.

10 Orlick T., Partington J. Excellence through mental training. *Sport Psychol Bull.* 1986; 69–75.

11 McDonald J., Orlick T., Letts M. Mental readiness in surgeons and its links to performance excellence in surgery. *J Bone Joint Surg A.* 1994.

12 Arora S., Aggarwal R., Moran A., Sirimanna P., et al. Mental practice: effective stress management training for novice surgeons. *J Am Coll Surg.* 2011; 212: 225–33.

13 Moran A. Cognitive psychology in sport: progress and prospects. *Psychol Sport Exerc.* 2009; 10(4): 420–6.

14 Schmidt R.A., Wrisberg C.A. *Motor Learning and Performance: a problem-based learning approach.* 3rd ed. Champaign, Illinois: Human Kinetics; 2004.

15 Jacobson E. Electrical measurements of neuromuscular states during mental activities. *Am J Physiol.* 1930; 91: 567–606.

16 Isaac A. Mental practice: does it work in the field? *Sport Psychol.* 1992; 6: 192–8.

17 Rodgers W., Hall C., Buckolz E. The effect of an imagery training program on imagery ability, imagery use, and skating performance. *J Appl Sport Psychol.* 1991; 3(2): 109–25.

18 Newell F.N., Ernst M.O., Tjan B.S., Buelthoff H.H. Viewpoint dependence in visual and haptic object recognition. *Psychol Sci.* 2001; 12(1): 37–42.

19 Kosslyn S.M., Ball T.M., Reiser B.J. Visual images preserve metric spatial information: evidenced from studies of image scanning. *J Exp Psychol Hum Percept Perform.* 1978; 4(1): 47–60.

20 Louis M., Guillot A., Maton S., Doyon J., Collet C. Effect of imagined movement speed on subsequent motor performance. *J Mot Behav.* 2008; 40(2): 117–32.

21 Jolly B. Clinical logbooks: recording clinical experiences may not be enough. *Med Educ.* 1999; 33(2): 86–8.

CHAPTER 10

Optimising surgical decisions and stress reduction

Good judgement and sound decision making have high standing as surgical attributes. Stress affects cognitive processes involving memory, recall of knowledge and attention. One of the most important effects of acute stress is on decision-making capacity. Although this capacity is just as important as operative skills, hardly any empirical information is available on the impact of stress on surgical decision making. This may be due to the fact that unlike technical skill, the impact of stress on decision making cannot be easily observed. The impact of your intraoperative decisions may be immediate and drastic. And the outcome of your decision may cause reduction in your stress or may worsen it!

Within other highly skilled, safety-critical industries like the military, evidence shows that stress has an effect on decision making by distracting attention from the primary task, disrupting the ability to use working memory, and by limiting the opportunity to gather enough information to make a decision. The whole persona of a surgeon is somebody who can make quick decisions and cope with anything. However, when things go wrong, a surgeon may not be able to think straight and so loses judgement, and everything descends into chaos.

How do surgeons make decisions under conditions of time pressure, increased risk, and when unexpected conditions or unanticipated problems emerge during the operation? This is not only relevant to emergency surgery; unforeseen conditions requiring new decisions and/or a change of plan may also occur in elective surgery. Imagine you are performing an endoscopy. You feel a little resistance while inserting the scope. You keep on inserting it further. A few second later, an enormous gush of blood blows out of the scope! You are in trouble. No guideline, no protocol, can help you in this situation. The only thing that can save you is your intuitive decision or what is called 'gut feeling' or instant reaction. For you to make optimum decisions in these situations, it is important to be aware of how we make decisions.

In recent years, changes in the configuration of surgical training have reduced the time spent by trainees in the operating theatre. The consequent reduction in attendance in the operating theatre produces a concomitant reduction in exposure to clinical situations. The loss of experience in making decisions, both in the operating theatre and during perioperative management, needs to be compensated for by improved teaching in decision making. To do this effectively, the cognitive processes used by surgeons need to be understood.

WHY GOOD SURGEONS MAKE BAD DECISIONS

Here is a true story depicted by Dr Jerome Groopman, Chair of Medicine at Harvard Medical School, in his book *How Doctors Think*.[1] Dr Groopman had been troubled by pain and swelling in his right hand for a few months. He consulted a hand surgeon – for the sake of confidentiality, it was Dr A. After the clinical examination and X-rays, Dr A could not find any abnormality apart from cysts in the scaphoid and lunate, which, according to him, were not related to the problem. He advised Dr Groopman to use a splint for a month. Despite using the splint, the symptoms persisted, and an MRI scan was carried out. Even this did not reveal any pathology apart from the cysts. Over the course of the following year, Dr Groopman had various other investigations, tried splinting again and had local steroid injections, without any improvement. Whenever Dr Groopman asked what was wrong with his wrist, Dr A could not offer a diagnosis. After undergoing treatment for a year without any benefit, Dr Groopman expressed his concerns, to which Dr A replied that Dr Groopman had developed 'hyperactive synovium' and needed surgery.

Not impressed by this unusual diagnosis and unclear treatment, Dr Groopman went to another orthopaedic surgeon – Dr B. At the outset, Dr B dismissed Dr A's diagnosis of 'hyperactive synovium' by remarking that such a term doesn't exist. When Dr B saw the X-rays and MRI he found not just a cyst, but also a hairline fracture in the scaphoid. Looking at the MRI, he recommended three separate surgical procedures. The first would pin the fracture, the second would drain the cysts and fill each of them with bone grafts, and the third would reposition the displaced tendon. He added that complete recovery might take up to 2 years.

Although Dr Groopman was desperate for relief, the idea of undergoing three operations spanning 2 years was not acceptable. He decided to consult a third surgeon, Dr C, one of the most renowned hand surgeons in the US. When Dr Groopman went to see Dr C, an assistant initially saw him. Dr C then came into the room and, while listening to the history from the assistant, examined Dr Groopman's hand. After a couple of minutes, he went to see the X-ray. He came back and advised him to have an arthroscopy. Not satisfied with this decision Dr Groopman asked him what he thought regarding a diagnosis. Dr C curtly replied that according to him he had 'chondrocalcinosis'. Dr Groopman, being a doctor himself, was conscious that nothing in any of the tests suggested chondrocalcinosis. He was also aware that, even if the diagnosis had been chondrocalcinosis, arthroscopy would not be of any help. Dr C had offered a diagnosis that, while not invented like Dr A's hyperactive synovium, was nevertheless unconvincing. Obviously Dr Groopman did not agree to the procedure.

A year later, when he could not bear the pain any longer, Dr Groopman went to a fourth orthopaedic surgeon, Dr D, who surprised Dr Groopman by examining not only his right hand, the symptomatic hand, but also the left one. Dr D X-rayed both hands, not only while the hands were stationary but also when they were in a gripping position. This was the first time anyone had ever paid attention to the left wrist or tried an X-ray of the hands during a manoeuvre. After looking at the X-rays, Dr D concluded that the ligaments between the bones were partially torn and that there were channels within the bone cysts and the joint, which were causing inflammation of the joint. When Dr Groopman mentioned that earlier MRIs had not revealed any of these problems, Dr D replied that, despite the negative MRI findings, he was confident that the ligaments were abnormal and that the connection existed between the cysts and the joints. According to him, surgeons relied too much on such sophisticated investigations; sometimes these had to be discounted if they were out of sync with the clinical picture. Dr D proposed taking a bone graft from the hip, filling in the cyst and repairing the ligaments in one operation.

Dr Groopman writes in *How Doctors Think* that over the course of 3 years he consulted many hand surgeons in the US and obtained as many different opinions about what was wrong and what to do, all the time continuing to suffer. One should not trivialise this case by saying, 'It happens – after all, people have different experiences'. It is disappointing to see that a Head of the Department of Medicine at Harvard could not get satisfactory treatment for his wrist pain in spite of consulting various surgeons over a period of 3 years. It needs to be stressed that the surgeons whom Dr Groopman consulted were well qualified and competent at their jobs. They had experience and an array of information at their fingertips. Their integrity or ability was not in doubt. But still, they did not get it right. One cannot dismiss this case by thinking of it as an aberration. It can happen to anybody and anywhere.

Decision making lies at the heart of our surgeons' professional lives. Every day we make decisions – decisions that affect patients' lives. Some are small, others more important. We make mistakes along the way. Indeed, the daunting reality is that important decisions made by intelligent, responsible professionals with the best information and intentions sometimes go wrong. Even good surgeons make bad decisions. How can we reduce the number of bad decisions that are made?

With all his experience with the orthopaedic surgeons he saw, Dr Groopman went to see Dr Terry Light, a former president of the American Orthopaedic Association. After listening to Dr Groopman's story, Dr Light said, 'The key is for everything to add up – the patient's symptoms, the findings on physical examination and investigations. It has to come together and form a coherent picture.' In effect, he was describing pattern recognition, and saying that if a clear pattern is not apparent, then the surgeon is in difficulty. Picking up a scalpel and cutting can be the wrong thing to do. Unfortunately, this is what Drs A, B and C, without recognising a coherent and consistent pattern, were set to do.

It is not that we are unaware of the uncertainties in surgical practice and have done nothing about it, because we have. We have attempted to address these uncertainties by various means, as mentioned before; we have enriched our knowledge and created an evidence base, among other things. But how far do you think surgical practice is evidence based? The majority of surgeons would like to answer by saying, 'Most of it'. However, that would not be an honest reply. Various studies reveal that surgeons do not practise evidence-based medicine as much as they would like to believe.[1] Dr Jack Weinberg has studied surgical decision making. What he has found is an embarrassing degree of inconsistency in the actions taken by surgeons.[2] His research has shown that the chance of a patient being advised to have a cholecystectomy varied by up to 70%, while recommendations for a hip replacement varied by up to 50%. This reflects the uncertainty in surgical practice, with the varied experience and attitudes of individual surgeons leading to massively different surgical management. Although the knowledge of what the right thing to do often exists, we still frequently fail to do it. Informed knowledge has simply not made its way far enough into actual practice. Overall, compliance with various evidence-based guidelines ranges from over 70% of patients in some studies to less than 20% in others. The grey areas in surgery are considerable. Every day we confront situations in which clear evidence of what to do is missing, and yet choices must be made. Exactly which patient suffering from back pain should be operated and which should be treated by conservative measures? For many cases, the answers can be obvious, but for many others we simply do not know. In the absence of evidence about what to do for a particular patient, you learn in surgery to make decisions based on your personal experience.

Here is a depiction of a conversation between three surgeons about a complication experienced by their colleague: a leak following an emergency sigmoid resection and primary anastomosis for sigmoid diverticulitis with contained contamination.

'Clearly,' said Dr Wilson, 'this was a serious lapse of judgement. I cannot imagine what he was thinking when he decided to put the colon back together again. He put his patient at risk unnecessarily.'

'I do not agree,' said Dr Lewis. 'There is good evidence that anastomosis can be performed safely on an unprepared bowel. This was a recognised complication, and simply reflects the fact that we will never eliminate complications entirely.'

'Maybe,' said Dr Smith, 'but data from experimental studies shows that faecal loading impairs anastomotic healing. The approach may be safe in ideal circumstances, but not in a man who has known co-morbidities. I would not have attempted an anastomosis here.'

'The point is,' said Dr Wilson, 'that, in the real world, patients are not experimental rats or carefully chosen subjects who are enrolled in clinical trials, but living, breathing humans who have plenty of associated health problems, who are operated on not by ultra-specialists in tertiary centres, but by surgeons like you and me. You do not take chances; you do the safest thing possible, and, for me, that would have been a Hartmann's procedure.'

Did the surgeon err in his judgement during the procedure? What would have been the safest course of action? What would have been best for the patient? Is there a right answer, and how can we ever know? Research has shown that a significant number of surgical complications is due to thinking errors rather than technical errors. Inappropriate decisions are made because of deviations in the thinking process. Biases sneak into our decision-making processes. They come out of our attempts to find short cuts. Most of us are busy in our day-to-day clinical work; our lives are stressful and we can't spend all our time thinking and analysing everything. When we have to make judgements, especially during a stressful operation, we use simple rules of thumb to help us make a decision. We use rules of thumb because, most of the time, they are quick and useful. In many cases, these short cuts are helpful. However, they can also lead to severe distortions of the thinking process. Some people learn the tricks to manage the thinking process. They know their biases and have figured out how to minimise their impact. The scientific term for a rule of thumb is a 'heuristic'. Heuristics are important contributors to experience and, to the uninitiated, they may appear to be trivial; for example, the use of packs to provide exposure, the use of tissue tension to facilitate dissection, and the way that fingers are used to expose a bleeding vessel.[3] These are short statements or actions that guide our thinking. One can say that heuristics are short statements drawn on long experience! Some heuristics are handed over to us by other experienced surgeons and some we develop from our own experience. Heuristics are methods of solving problems when no formula exists. Such tricks of the trade are informal and are based on experience. They are informal because iteration, such as the repeated performance of an operation, results in the unconscious development of techniques for overcoming problems. All experienced surgeons have such traits and they collectively contribute to an operating style. Risk management cannot advance without a genuine understanding of how surgeons work, and this requires a greater appreciation of heuristics. The mental heuristics that experienced surgeons use to minimise risk are usually expressed in the form of anecdotes. This is why informal talk between operations and in the lifts and corridors during rounds is so important; it helps to socialise trainees into the profession of surgery.

INTUITIVE DECISIONS: DOES IT MAKE (SIXTH) SENSE?

Although surgeons have not taken the decision-making skill seriously, others have. Here is a story from the first Gulf war in 1991, when coalition warships were deployed off the Kuwaiti coast.[4] Lieutenant Commander Michael Riley was monitoring the radar screens on board HMS *Gloucester*, a British warship. The ship was responsible for protecting the coalition fleet. At 5 o'clock in the morning, he noticed a radar blip off the Kuwaiti coast. A quick calculation of its trajectory had it heading for the convoy. Although Riley had been staring at similar blips all night long, there was something about this radar trace that immediately made him suspicious. He couldn't explain why, but the blinking green dot on the screen filled him with apprehension. He continued to observe the incoming blip for another 40 seconds as it slowly honed in on the USS *Missouri*, an American warship. It was approaching the American ship at more than 500 miles per hour. If Riley was going to shoot down the target – if he was going to act on his fear – then he needed to respond right away. If Riley did not move immediately, it would be too late. The USS *Missouri* would be sunk and Riley would have stood by and watched it happen.

But Riley had a problem. The radar blip was located in airspace that was frequently used by American fighter jets. The blip was travelling at the same speed as the fighter jets. It looked exactly like an A6 on the radar screen. To make matters even more complicated, the A6 pilots had got into the habit of turning off their electronic identification on their return flights. As a result, the radar crew on board HMS *Gloucester* had no way of contacting them.

The target was moving fast. Riley issued the order to fire; two Sea Dart surface-to-air missiles were launched. Soon an explosion echoed over the ocean. The captain of HMS *Gloucester* asked Riley how he could be sure he had fired at an Iraqi missile and not an American fighter jet. Riley said: 'I just knew.'

Every surgeon must be familiar with the feeling of 'I just knew'. There are many actions surgeons take that they find difficult to explain. In the early days of training, you might have observed an experienced surgeon making a diagnosis of a very complex case just by history and examination. If anybody had asked him how he reached his decision, he might have said, 'I just knew.' Some call it experience, while others say it is intuition. Decision science calls it 'System 1 thinking'.

The next four hours were the longest of Riley's life. If he had shot down an A6, he had killed two innocent pilots, and his career was over. After a four-hour wait, the captain of HMS *Gloucester* was informed that the radar blip was, in fact, a Silkworm missile, and not an American fighter jet. Riley had single-handedly saved a warship.

After the war was over, British naval officers analysed the events preceding Riley's decision to fire the Sea Dart missiles. They concluded that, with the information available to Lieutenant Commander Riley, it was impossible for him to distinguish between the Silkworm and a friendly A6. Although Riley had made the correct decision, he could just as easily have been shooting down an American fighter jet. His risky gamble paid off, but it had still been a gamble.

That, at least, was the official version of events until Gary Klein, a cognitive psychologist, got involved. He proved that it was nothing like a gamble. Gary soon realised that Riley had become accustomed to seeing very consistent blip patterns when A6s returned from their bombing sorties. The planes typically became visible after a single radar sweep. Klein analysed the radar tapes from the predawn missile attack. He replayed those fateful 40 seconds over and over again, searching for any differences between Riley's experience of A6s returning from their sorties and his experience of the Silkworm blip. Klein suddenly saw the discrepancy. It was subtle, but crystal clear. He could finally explain Riley's thought process. The secret was timing. Unlike the A6, the Silkworm did not appear off the coast right away. Because it travelled at such a low altitude – nearly 2000 feet below an A6 – the signal of the missile was initially masked by ground interference. As a result, it was not visible until the third radar sweep, which was eight seconds after an A6 would have appeared. Riley was unconsciously evaluating the altitude of the blip, even if he did not know he was.

This is why Riley got the chills when he stared at the Iraqi missile on his radar screen. There was something strange about the radar blip. It did not feel like an A6. Although Riley could not explain why he felt so scared, he knew that something scary was happening. This blip needed to be shot down.

There are two reasons for mentioning this story here: first, to get interesting accounts of intuitive decision making during a critical situation;

and, second, to show how other professionals are taking intuitive decision making seriously. The military has taken intuitive decision making to a formal level. The US military has incorporated intuitive decision making in its training programme. This has been a massive change for an organisation that is run on strict rules and procedures.

Although it has been known for a long time that surgeons use intuitive thinking, especially during critical and stressful situations, it has not been given serious consideration. We hardly know anything about it. If we have any problems due to the process of intuitive thinking, the first step is to know what it entails.

Conventional methods of surgical practice and surgical training are becoming outdated. Unless we make conscious efforts to sharpen our intuitive skills, we may not be able to perform effectively and efficiently in stressful situations. Guidelines and protocols have a certain place in management. They can be useful for run-of-the-mill diagnoses and treatment. But they quickly fall apart when you need to think outside the box, and when symptoms are vague or multiple and the investigations are inconclusive. To manage these kinds of cases, you need discerning thinking. Protocols unfortunately discourage people from thinking independently and creatively. Instead of expanding clinicians' thinking, they can restrain it.

There are a lot of misconceptions about intuitive decision making. There are individuals who are intolerant towards the idea of making a decision with intuitive thinking. According to Benner, '… intuition is the black-market version of the knowledge'.[5] People may not realise the disadvantage they incur due to their attitude. They may not be aware that you may not trust intuition, but you cannot survive without it. Unfortunately, we have not taken a scientific approach towards this wonderful faculty. Similar to other scientific developments, cognitive science has progressed over the last few years. It would be unwise to remain fixated on the traditional view of intuition.

So what exactly happens when you take an intuitive decision about your patient? To get the answer, think about the times when you had a sense about something, even though you couldn't quite explain it. What is it that sets off the alarm bells inside your head when apparently the case appears to be 'just a routine one'? It is an intuition, built up through repeated experiences that you have unconsciously linked together to form a pattern. That's how we have hunches about what is really going on and about what we should do.

The more patterns we learn, the easier it is to match a new situation to one of the patterns in your reservoir. When a new situation occurs, we recognise the situation as familiar by matching it to a pattern we have encountered in the past. Once we recognise a pattern, we gain a sense of situation: we know what cues are going to be important and need to be monitored. We have a sense of what to expect next. And the patterns include routines for responding. If we see a situation as typical, we can recognise the typical ways to react.

The following think-aloud will illustrate intuition in a surgical context.[6] Here, a surgeon is asked to put across his views about the management of a patient.

Q A 16-year-old girl reports right lower quadrant (RLQ) pain for 6 hours and mild RLQ tenderness. Temperature: 37°C. No nausea or vomiting. She is in the mid-cycle of her menstrual period. WBC: 7800. No shift. What are your thoughts?

A You are always worried about appendicitis, but it's early in the course of events. People usually don't have to worry about a ruptured appendix for 24–36 hours. If you don't think she has surgical indications, it's probably safe to watch her. It sounds like she probably has mittelschmerz because she is mid-cycle in her period; assuming she is not on birth-control pills. You need to know if she is hungry or not, and if she typically has such pain during her cycle. You also need to do a pelvic exam. I wouldn't operate on her at this point.

Q An ultrasound of the pelvis shows a slight amount of fluid in the cul-de-sac but is otherwise normal.

A Same thing – she could have a ruptured cyst, and they didn't see it.

Q The pain persists overnight. Tenderness in the RLQ persists. The on-call surgeon performs laparoscopy. Tubes, ovaries and appendix are normal. What would you do in this situation?

A Appendix, tubes and ovaries are normal. I would probably do a laparoscopic appendectomy while I was there, but I would not do anything further.

Q What triggers an operation for possible appendicitis? What does not trigger it?

A   I think the single most important thing is how tender the patient is over the appendix, in association with a compatible history. What does not trigger me to operate on appendicitis? Early in the course, less than 6 hours, less than 24 hours, I am not as worried. White blood cell counts don't help me very much. Patients who are hungry usually don't have appendicitis. A lot of people say they are hungry, but I think only once in my life have I had a patient with appendicitis who wanted to go to McDonald's for a Big Mac and fries, which is my standard question. They frequently say, 'Sure, I'm hungry,' and I say, 'You want a Big Mac and fries at McDonald's?' and they go, 'Uh, I don't think so.' It's a rare patient who is hungry. I am inclined not to jump on them if it's particularly early in the course and the situation is confusing. But the most important determining factor is how tender the patient is over the appendix. In a patient with localised tenderness and significant guarding who is over 24 hours out, I simply take out the appendix. It's a clinical decision.

This case illustrates how we use intuition in a routine surgical case. This surgeon's thoughts concerning whether to operate for suspected appendicitis are an example of intuitive judgement. The surgeon pays attention to several factors simultaneously – amount and location of tenderness, duration of symptoms, appetite – and bases the decision on them. He cannot verbalise the rules governing the decision precisely. Judgements of this type have several features that differentiate them from analytical thinking. First, the result of the judgement is one of three possible actions: send the patient home, wait and see what develops, or operate. Second, several features have a bearing on the judgement, such as the patient's sex, age and weight. Also relevant are features of the present illness, such as location, intensity and quality of the right lower quadrant pain, as well as the patient's appetite. But it is not just the current state of these variables that is important: the surgeon also pays attention to how they have varied over the past few hours and days. These variables actually make the decision even simpler, for they allow the surgeon to focus on just two actions: send home versus wait, or wait versus operate. Of course, as the situation changes, the surgeon may focus on a different pair of options, but at any one moment the decision is simply between two alternatives. A third feature of such judgements is that the experts do not know exactly how they make them. They can say sensible things about each feature, such as, 'If the patient has an appetite, it is probably not appendicitis,' but they cannot say how the various features are combined into their overall sense of whether they should operate.

Intuition is the way we translate our experiences into decisions. It is that ability to make decisions by using patterns to recognise what is going on in a situation and to recognise the typical action plan with which to react. Once an experienced intuitive decision maker sees the pattern, any decision she has to make is usually obvious.

A pattern is a set of features that usually chunk together so that if you see a few of the features you can expect to find the others. When you notice a pattern, you have a sense of familiarity – yes, I have seen it before! As we work in our particular professional field, we accumulate experiences and build up a reservoir of recognised patterns. The more patterns and action plans we have available, the more expertise we have, and the easier it is to make decisions. Without the repertoire of patterns and action scripts, we would have to painstakingly think out every situation from scratch. Because pattern matching can take place in an instant, and without conscious thought, we are not aware of how we arrived at an intuitive judgement. That is why it often seems mysterious to us. Even if the situation isn't exactly the same as anything we have seen before, we can recognise similarities with past events and so we automatically know what to do, without having to deliberately think out the options. We have a sense of what will work and what won't.

The other, rather interesting, way to describe intuition is to say it's a joke. To be specific, it is like a joke. When you listen to a joke, you find it funny. The joke is funny only if you get it. And you get it instantly, like a flash. If you don't get the joke and if somebody explains it you, it loses the punch and the fun. The instant appreciation of a joke is equivalent to instant recognition by intuition. Just as some people lack a sense of humour, some people do not develop an intuitive sense. On the other hand, like some 'very funny' people, some have a strong intuitive sense. To complete the analogies, for you to get the joke you need to know the background and context of the joke. The same is true of intuition. You need to know the context of a clinical situation to make an intuitive decision.

Here is another case given to a neurosurgeon.[6]

Q You have gone to see an American football match at your local club. A 16-year-old football player becomes unconscious for 30 seconds, and then walks to the sidelines. You are called to the sidelines to see him. How would you examine him? What would you do?

A I am assuming that the mechanism was not a fall while he was running for a pass by himself. That suggests subarachnoid haemorrhage, like a spontaneous bleed into a brain tumour, although such a mechanism is unlikely in a 16 year old. It's not going to be diffuse axonal injury for two reasons: number one, he got up and walked to the sidelines; and the second reason is the diffuse axonal injury is a big mechanism. So it isn't going to be a diffuse axonal injury, because the mechanism is not right. The mechanism is right for a contusion of the brain. The chance of a subdural haematoma is very small, because first, the mechanism is not right, and second, he's too young. The possibility of epidural haematoma is also very small. You need a skull fracture. How many times do you fracture a skull with a helmet on? Rarely. So you're probably looking at a contusion, possibly as minor as a concussion.

Q How would you manage him?

A I'd look at three things: level of consciousness, pupillary exam, and best motor response.

Q He is awake and alert. Pupillary exam is normal. Motor exam is normal as well; he can jog up and down the field.

A He sits out for at least 5 or 6 minutes. Has his neurological exam changed?

Q No, it has not changed.

A Then the question is, 'Is he laying down any new information? Does he know what the score is?'

Q He is a little fuzzy on what happened to him.

A Then he doesn't go back in.

Q He doesn't go back in the game? Does he go to the hospital?

A If he gets any worse, he goes to the hospital immediately. He should only get better from the moment of impact, not worse.

Q You examine him and you talk to him. He is really fuzzy and doesn't know what is going on. He complains of a mild headache. You send him to the hospital. Does he have to have a CT scan?

A When he gets to the hospital, has he got any worse?

Q He still has retrograde amnesia and keeps repeating the same question: 'What happened to me? What happened to me?' But beyond that he is okay.

A In that case, he would get a CT scan.

Q I notice you didn't look in his fundi.

A No. That wastes time.

Q Why? Doesn't it help you?

A No. You know what his neurological exam is. You know exactly how his whole brain is functioning.

Q You don't need a reflex hammer?

A I don't need a reflex hammer. You see how you have to take the situation of your practice into account.

PATTERN RECOGNITION

Have you noticed in this think-aloud how the neurosurgeon recognised and focused on key elements of the case? His thinking is efficient for various reasons. In addition to the knowledge, which is well organised for rapid access, the surgeon also knows what is important and can focus on the key elements of the case.

Thus, when initially engaged in pattern recognition, the surgeon knows to pay attention to the mechanism of the injury – a tackle involves more force than a spontaneous bleed into a brain tumour, but less than would produce a diffuse axonal injury. Large numbers of possibilities are eliminated through the use of one, highly diagnostic, cue.

Later, he focuses on any changes in the football player's ability to think. Because the boy can reveal his state of consciousness, any more detailed neurological exam would be redundant. Any deterioration in his awareness would make the surgeon send him to the hospital.

Expert clinicians condense a case into manageable form, focusing on one or two pivotal findings. Success with this strategy depends, of course, on being able to judge which of many possible features of the case to focus on.

VISUALISATION IN SURGICAL DECISION MAKING[6]

Q A 30-year-old woman had a laparoscopic cholecystectomy for acute cholecystitis 6 weeks previously. She is now jaundiced with a bilirubin of 14 and alkaline phosphates of 350. AST and ALT are normal. What are your thoughts? What work-up would you use?

A You would have to be concerned that you either injured her common duct or left behind a stone in the bile duct. She needs endoscopic retrograde cholangiopancreatography (ERCP) as the next step, which would be diagnostic and potentially therapeutic.

Q They are unable to do an ERCP. What will you do now?

A I would do a transhepatic cholangiogram in an attempt to define where the problem was. Then she will have to have an operation.

Q A percutaneous transhepatic cholangiogram shows several clips at the area of the cystic duct stump with a 0.5 cm narrowing of the common duct adjacent to the clips. What do you do?

A I am trying to visualise what you just told me. You would have to assume a duct injury. I think I would operate on the patient.

Q Describe what you would do in the operation.

A You have to figure out what is wrong. The patient has developed a stricture. You probably have a common duct injury from the procedure itself. It may be as simple as the fact that you put the clips too close to the common bile duct, and you may be able to alleviate the problem by removing them and closing over the cystic duct. If the duct has been significantly injured, like cut in two, it will have to be repaired, probably with a Roux-en-Y choledochojejunostomy as opposed to a direct repair by putting the two ends of the duct together. It's hard for me to visualise the problem, but you have to find out what's wrong, and you have to operate to do it. Then you have to make the appropriate repair.

Given a description of postoperative complications, the surgeon tries to visualise what went wrong. He would prefer ERCP, with its superior visualisation and the possibility of inserting instruments, to the static image of the cholangiogram. If it was his own operation, he also might 'rewind the video tape', recalling the operation to see if any details of the procedure could explain what is happening now. Given a verbal description of the results of the cholangiogram, the surgeon needs time to visualise them, to create an image of the patient's organs after the cholecystectomy. Knowledge from a variety of sources goes into this visualisation: knowledge of the normal anatomy of the organs, the disease that led to the original operation and the typical efficacy of that operation, and the procedures used when the gall bladder is removed via laparoscope, as opposed to an open operation. It takes time to construct a full visualisation. This is not due just to the fact that the surgeon was not offered an X-ray, for it takes time to interpret an X-ray image too. The surgeon did not get a complete picture of exactly what had happened, but could assume it was a duct injury and that an operation is therefore necessary.

DECISION DEPENDS ON PATTERN RECOGNITION[6]

Q A 55-year-old man presents with gross melaena. Four units of blood are required to restore his blood pressure to normal. Endoscopy demonstrates a posterior duodenal ulcer with an oozing vessel in the base. What are your thoughts?

A If the duodenum is terribly scarred and you had to do a resection to get at it, I would insert a tube duodenostomy and close it. This procedure always works to keep you out of trouble in an emergency situation.

Q On the fifth postoperative day the patient is jaundiced with a bilirubin of 8 and an alkaline phosphatase of 300; the other liver enzymes are normal. What would you do?

A The patient needs endoscopic retrograde cholangiopancreatography (ERCP) or a percutaneous transhepatic cholangiogram to make sure that I did not injure his common bile duct with my sutures. I would think back over exactly what I did, suture wise, at the operation and see if I feasibly could have put a suture around the common duct.

Q On the seventh postoperative day, the patient vomits a large amount of blood. What would you do?

A I would repeat the endoscopy if at all possible. The patient could be bleeding from the suture line. I would keep in mind that the gastroenterologist can sometimes zap something and save the patient an operation. I would re-operate if they couldn't figure it out or if he was bleeding profusely.

The surgeon rapidly recognises and responds to the situation. The elements of good decisions are present in these responses, although it is not easy to see them because the responses take place so quickly.

To make good decisions, one must know the options. In this think-aloud, the surgeon comes up with appropriate options. If the situation were different, different options would come to mind. One of the features of the human memory is that ideas come to mind when they are likely to be needed.

The surgeon must also know what can happen. Examples in the think-aloud include the surgeon's comment on the tube duodenostomy, that it can 'keep you out of trouble', and his hypotheses about how he may have caused the postoperative jaundice by injuring the common bile duct with sutures.

A third aspect of careful thought about decisions is awareness of how likely various events are. The more likely causes and effects come quickly to the surgeon's mind – for example, the scarred duodenum and the bleeding from the suture line.

Decisions must also take into account how good or bad the results of one's actions can be. Such considerations are evident in this surgeon's script, as when he mentions the possibility of stemming the bleeding through the endoscope and thus saving the patient an operation.

Intuition is an important asset for all of us. Nevertheless, some people have difficulty in acknowledging that we use experience in this way, and some have trouble explaining the basis of their reasoning when someone else asks them to defend their judgements. Therefore, intuition has a bad reputation compared with judgement that comes from careful analysis. However, research[7] has shown that people do worse at some decision tasks when they are asked to perform analysis of the reason for their preference or evaluate the attributes of the different choices. This will especially apply to the decisions made in the operating theatre.

Intuition is not perfect. Our experience will sometimes mislead us, and we will make mistakes that add to our experience base. Imagine that you're driving around in an unfamiliar city, and you see some landmark, perhaps a petrol pump, and you say, 'Oh, now I know where we are,' and (despite the protests of your spouse, who has the map) make a fateful turn and wind up on an inescapable entrance to the motorway that you had been trying to avoid. As you face the prospect of being sent miles out of your way, you may lamely offer that the petrol pump you remembered must have been a different one: 'I thought I recognised it, but I guess I was wrong.'

The next think-aloud, by surgeons at four different levels of experience, makes it very easy to see the progression in the ideas that the surgeons bring to the case. We can see differences in what the surgeons recognise and in the strategies they use.[6]

Q A 65-year-old obese man, who is a known alcoholic, presents to A&E with a two-year history of severe epigastric abdominal pain. His BP is 200/110, pulse is 110 per minute, and his stool is positive for occult blood.

Junior grade resident: I am very concerned about his abdominal pain and his tachycardia. I am worried that he has intra-abdominal bleeding of some kind. I would like to know how long he has had the abdominal pain.

Middle grade resident: First of all, you have to instigate resuscitation. Then you begin your investigation to determine the nature of his abdominal pain. Basic laboratory tests should be ordered, chest X-ray, KUB. Specifically, you entertain diagnoses such as duodenal ulcer, perforated or not, some sort of gastric problem, problems associated with the history of alcoholism and potentially a history of blood clot.

Senior grade resident: I first thought of an ulcer disease or some other alcohol-related duodenal or gastric process, but, in the back of my mind, I think that I need to rule out something separate from the alcohol disease, like an abdominal aortic aneurysm, especially in view of the epigastric pain. With the positive occult blood in stool, I think of an ulcer and something going along with that. I want to know if he has been vomiting and what that would show. I would like to get more information about related symptoms.

Attending surgeon: Obese, alcoholic male with epigastric pain and positive occult blood in stool. I am going to start IVs and get some baseline laboratory data and a CT scan. I certainly want a full blood count to see whether he has lost a significant amount of blood.

Maybe, baseline liver-function tests and an X-ray of his chest. I am thinking, epigastric pain in an alcoholic male: gastritis, perforated ulcer. Biliary tract is unlikely.

Q The patient has the IIb of 9, an arterial pO2 of 7.25, a pCO2 of 80, and a base deficit of 10. Abdominal ultrasound in A&E is non-diagnostic because of obesity. His ECG shows sinus tachycardia, his LFTs are within normal range, his BP is 100 and his pulse is 120.

Junior grade resident: The patient is acidotic, and so far that is the only abnormal test result I know about. His blood pressure is dropping, and I am still very concerned about the abdominal bleeding.

Middle grade resident: We have not established a diagnosis yet. The patient is acidotic. His BP continues to drop and he is becoming more tachycardic despite the resuscitation. Therefore, I would consider some sort of intra-abdominal catastrophe. A few critical pieces of information are still missing.

Senior grade resident: It sounds like a perforated duodenal ulcer. Since he is acidotic, he is going into shock.

Attending surgeon: I would do an abdominal examination to see if he is tender anywhere. I would put in an NG tube to see if we are really dealing with upper GI bleeding. Pain plus a drop in BP might mean a ruptured aneurysm. CT could help. I don't think an upper GI endoscopy is going to help.

Q A CT scan is done, which confirms a 6 cm abdominal aortic aneurysm.

Junior grade resident: He needs an operation.

Middle grade resident: He needs to be taken to theatre.

Senior grade resident: We are going to operate.

Attending surgeon: I don't think we have much time to mess around. We are heading towards the operating room.

The ideas that come to mind become both more detailed and more focused as one gains experience. The junior surgical trainee, who saw abdominal pain and low blood pressure, worried about intra-abdominal bleeding. This, of course, is correct, but non-specific. The others show more specific ideas. They look for particular observations or test results and have more specific explanations for the patient's symptoms. The junior trainee is still trying to figure out what to notice, whereas the more experienced residents usually notice the right facts but still have to figure out what to do with them.

Both the senior grade resident and the attending surgeon considered the possibility of an abdominal aortic aneurysm before it was reported in the CT scan results. They mentioned it at different times. The senior grade resident mentioned it after the first description of the patient as part of his broad initial response. The attending surgeon mentioned it after receiving the laboratory tests and hearing of the sudden drop in blood pressure. For the senior grade resident, it was a general rule: 'If an alcoholic presents with belly pain, rule out abdominal aortic aneurysm before assuming ulcer.' For the attending, it was a more specific recognition: 'Pain plus drop in blood pressure may mean ruptured aneurysm.' The difference between the two is a sign of 'tuning' one's knowledge. The attending surgeon's mind works more efficiently, applying hypotheses when they are most likely to be needed, and not bothering to consider them explicitly when there is not yet sufficient reason to do so.

When you don't have a well-tuned script that enables you to recognise automatically the key features of the situation, to identify the important hypotheses, and to respond appropriately, you have to figure out the situation logically. In this kind of problem solving, rules of thumb can be helpful. As one gains experience, the rules become more specific, as befits more specific knowledge.

Thus, the junior grade resident guides her thinking with a very general rule: 'Pay attention to what brought the patient in.' This rule orients her to the need to find out all the facts, yet reminds her not to become distracted by aspects of the patient's history that are unrelated to the present illness. The senior resident also uses a rule: 'Don't get fooled by the most obvious hypothesis', which reminds him to keep other hypotheses in mind and to look for opportunities to rule them out. Even though this general rule helped him to state the correct hypothesis of abdominal aortic aneurysm early in his thinking, the observation of the drop in blood pressure did not return his attention to it. At that point the attending surgeon recognised the correct hypothesis, although she had not explicitly put it on her initial list.

HOW DO THEY DO IT? EXPERT DECISION MAKING IN A STRESSFUL SITUATION

A foetus was diagnosed as having a large cystic hygroma.[8] The ultra-sonography showed that the hygroma had grown inside the neck, wrapping around the trachea. There was a risk of the infant being unable to breathe after the delivery. A Caesarean section was scheduled for the following day. During the delivery, the doctor in charge was going to determine if the baby was able to breathe on his own. If the baby could not, he was planning to intubate. If he was unable to intubate, he planned to do a tracheostomy, which would be a difficult procedure as the cystic hygroma was filling the space between the trachea and the skin. Upon delivery, the infant gave a cry, suggesting patent trachea. But after the cry the infant could not even grunt. The nurse suctioned the infant's mouth and placed him in front of the doctor.

The doctor remembered an earlier situation, when he had been called in to operate on a young man who had run his motorbike into a strand of barbed wire. The wire had jumbled the victim's neck tissue into sausage-like chunks. On that occasion, the paramedic had inserted an endotracheal tube. When the doctor wondered how this was done, the paramedic later explained that she stuck the tube where she saw bubbles. Bubbles meant air coming out of the trachea.

So, in the delivery room, the doctor looked into the mouth of the infant for bubbles. All he saw was a mass of yellow cysts, completely obscuring the vocal cords. No bubbles. What the doctor did was place his palm on the infant's chest and press down, to force the last bit of air out of the infant's lungs. The doctor saw a few tiny bubbles of saliva between some of the cysts and inserted the tube into that area. The infant quickly changed colour. The procedure had worked.

This case involved high-pressure problem solving by intuitive thinking. The doctor did not have any established procedure for inserting the endotracheal tube into the infant in such a situation. He recalled an analogous case – and a far-fetched one at that. It was about someone else's action, not his own. The key point of similarity was discovering the air passage in an obscured throat. And even the analogy was not sufficient. There were no bubbles. The doctor had to invent his own way to produce bubbles.

This kind of skilful problem solving is impressive because, after the fact, the solution seems obvious, yet we know that, without any guidance, in stressful situation like this, many would miss the answer. They would not even know that an answer was possible. We would look into the infant's mouth, see the mass of cysts, and abandon the idea of intubation, immediately resorting to tracheostomy.

Just as we are impressed when someone with expertise seems to know just what to do in a difficult situation, we are also impressed when someone invents a new procedure on the spot. Experts use intuitive thinking to create a new course of action, to notice something that may cause a difficulty before there are any obvious signs of trouble, and to figure out what is causing the difficulty.

EXPERT THINKING

Whenever senior surgeons make a difficult decision in a stressful situation that nobody else thought of, we give credit to their experience and say, 'Experience counts.' But merely saying that the surgeons used their experience is not sufficient. The useful thing is to find out how that experience came into play. The general belief is that logical thinking helps the experienced surgeon to make good decisions. However, if you assess the expert surgeons' thought process, you will realise that a significant portion of their thinking is not analytical, but intuitive. Intuitively, they are able to size up the clinical situation quickly and imagine how a course of action might be carried out; they also draw upon their experience by suggesting parallels between the current situation and something else that they had encountered before. We do not make someone an expert just through training him/her in analytical thinking. Quite the contrary is true – if we do that, we run the risk of slowing the development of decision-making skills.

Experts see the clinical situation and match it with their experience. When they start getting initial information, their brain begins to predict what other information they should expect to confirm the pattern. They pick up cues if particular information is missing or there is some information that shouldn't be there. One of Arthur Conan Doyle's stories shows how Sherlock Holmes solved a case using his ability to notice what did not happen. In 'Silver Blaze', the vital clue was a dog that did not bark at night. The dog usually barked when strangers went by. The fact that the murderer passed the dog in silence meant that the dog recognised him.

Experts appear to have an overall sense of what is happening in a situation. Whereas novices may be confused by all the information, experts see the big picture and appear to be less likely to fall victim to information overload. Also, when we see experts performing a surgical procedure, they appear smooth and neat. The reason for the smoothness is the detailed knowledge experts have about the procedure. They know not only the bigger picture, but also the smaller steps that constitute the whole procedure.

One of the ways of making decisions is to seek additional information. This may seem like a routine activity, but it also requires expertise. A mindless information-gathering strategy is unlikely to be useful. Experienced decision makers are able to spot circumstances and opportunities in which the information that can be helpful can be readily obtained. Skilled decision makers may be able to seek information more effectively than novices. This skill in information seeking would result in a more efficient search for data that clarifies the status of the situation.

Experts in any field can detect differences that novices cannot see, and cannot even force themselves to see. Wine tasters can tell one type of grape from another and even the year of the wine from another. To novices, wines are generic; they all taste the same. If you are just starting to drink wine, no matter how much attention you pay, and how much you swirl the fluid around in your mouth, you don't get it. That is because 'it' is not a fact or an insight. You cannot learn just by being told and you cannot learn all of a sudden. It takes experience, and lots of variety in that experience, to notice the difference.

An important part of expert development is that experts engage in deliberate practice. For them, each opportunity for practice has a goal and evaluation criteria. Mere accumulation of experiences is not sufficient. Experiences need to include feedback that is accurate and timely. In a domain where obtaining timely feedback is not possible, mere accumulation of experience does not result in the growth of expertise. Experts obtain feedback that is accurate and reasonably timely. They enrich their experience by reviewing prior experiences to develop insight and learn lessons from mistakes. In order to perform deliberate practice, people must articulate goals and identify the type of decisions they need to improve.

IMPROVING DECISIONS AND AVOIDING STRESSFUL SITUATIONS

Since we know that we rely on intuition for good-quality decisions, anybody who is keen to improve their decision making needs to develop intuition into a reliable tool. This is especially true in the context of decision making in stressful situations. Appropriate decisions will relieve you from stress while inappropriate decisions will worsen it. We need to treat intuitions as skills that can be acquired like any other skill. Expert surgeons don't just develop good judgement skills, any more than an athlete suddenly has an excellent day on the track. If you are working out for months at 15 minutes per mile, you are unlikely to sprint 7 minutes per mile within a day. This kind of improvement takes effort. Similarly, the kind of judgement that skilled surgeons make also takes work. They have to build up an experience base that lets them accurately size up situations. As with physical exercise, you could get strength by repetitions, but you will get better results if you use an appropriate strategy. In the same way, instead of passively waiting to acquire intuition through routine work, there are methods one can use to speed up the process. One of the methods is to develop the skill of blending intuition with analysis, and another is 'cognitive autopsy' or post-mortem of the decision-making process. For some surgeons, these techniques may be quite obvious. They wonder why such a big deal is made about it. The truth, however, is that it is not obvious to everyone. Even those who understand the importance of intuition do not adopt strategies to achieve good-quality intuition.

Trainees need to make efforts to develop their intuition. The challenge for them is to build intuitive decision-making skills as quickly as possible. We do not get any explicit guidance on developing intuition. As a result, you may flounder, get frustrated, and acquire bad habits and a poor attitude. The higher one goes in a surgical career, the greater the need for intuition. To develop good intuition, one needs to have a collection of various patterns. To develop a range of patterns, we need to get experience. Not every experience is useful for developing intuition. It should be a meaningful experience, an experience that allows us to recognise a pattern and use that pattern as a template for future reference. We think that day-to-day clinical experience is the most meaningful experience. Not necessarily. There are a few problems if you rely solely on clinical experience as a meaningful experience. First of all, getting the satisfactory meaningful experience depends upon chance and circumstances:

getting the appropriate job, being supervised by an appropriate surgeon, and so on. Also, the problem with relying on clinical experience is the time required to receive enough experience. It is said that it takes at least 10 years to become an expert in any field. With the changes happening in surgical training, surgeons would be expected to develop expertise in a shorter duration. Thus, gaining a meaningful real-life experience is not easy. We need to develop some other ways to seek meaningful experiences. In fact, developing alternative ways to acquire intuitive skills may prove better in some aspects. This is because it would involve 'deliberate practice'. Deliberate practice means not just practising to practise, gathering experience randomly, but practising with specific objectives in mind. Research has shown that meaningful experience and deliberate practice are the most vital ingredients for developing expertise.

PROBLEMS OF ANALYTICAL THINKING

If we asked anybody what the right way to make an important decision was, we would be told to analyse the problem thoroughly, evaluate all the options, and compare them to see which one was the best. This is a standard method of decision making and there is something appealing about it. It is based not on whims, but on solid analysis. It is methodical rather than haphazard. It guarantees that you won't miss anything important. It promises you a good decision if you follow the process properly. It allows you to justify your decision to others. It sounds reassuring. Who would not want to be thorough, systematic and scientific? *But*, there is a problem. The problem is that the whole thing becomes a myth in situations where it matters most: in a critical step of a case, a complex patient with many co-morbidities, unexpected finding during the procedure and so on. The reality is that analytical method does not always work well in practice. It works tolerably well on paper, but does not necessarily work in day-to-day clinical life, where decisions are more challenging, situations are more confusing and complex, information is scarce or inconclusive, time is short, and stakes are high. In these environments, the standard method of decision making may fall flat.

Nobody would disagree that, without rational analysis, we would not have the exciting growth in science and technology and progress in medicine. Decision trees and cost-benefit analysis can help us make sense of choices, but there are limitations. Just because these methods work in some situations, it does not mean that they work for all practical problems.

Not knowing the problems of this type of thinking, some people take rational thinking to the extreme. They turn out to be hyper-rational. When people become hyper-rational, they attempt to handle all problems, relying only on analytical reasoning. In the initial states, this can be (mis)perceived as a positive sign of critical thinking. Only later do we see an unwillingness to act without a rigid protocol. There is disregard for the needs of individual patients. They even lose common sense. If the problem is not checked in time, the final stages degenerate into what is called as 'paralysis by analysis'. A surgeon just sits on a case, when others would have intervened. To get an idea of how bad the problem of hyper-rationality is, consider two different kinds of ophthalmic diagnoses. One is macular degeneration, in which the fovea and the central zone of the retina are destroyed. The second is retinitis pigmentosa, in which the peripheral vision deteriorates. As we know, the fovea is the only part that is capable of fine discrimination. One may think that macular degeneration could be the worst visual impairment. Retinitis pigmentosa gives the impression of being less devastating than macular degeneration. But the reality is altogether different. Retinitis pigmentosa is a far more disorientating condition than macular degeneration. If you lost all your peripheral vision, you would have a tiny searchlight sweeping endlessly back and forth, trying to locate everything and retain orientation. Without peripheral vision, you would even have trouble sitting quietly and reading, since you need peripheral vision to direct your eye movements. Hyper-rationality is like retinitis pigmentosa, in which we try to do all our thinking with analysis. Rational thinking is like foveal vision using cone cells, which provides us with the ability to make fine discrimination but is not sufficient to maintain orientation, and is irrelevant during night-time. We need peripheral vision to detect where to apply the analysis and calculations.

Although problems with analytical thinking have been mentioned, we need to be aware that intuition cannot solve every problem. Analysis has a proper role as a supporting tool for making intuitive decisions. When time and the necessary information are available, analysis can help uncover cues and patterns. It can sometimes help evaluate a decision. But it cannot replace the intuition that is at the centre of the decision-making process, although that is precisely what some people try to do. We are advised to suppress our intuitions, because, as we are told, intuitions are inherently biased. One can agree that we shouldn't blindly follow all intuitions, as they can be unreliable and need to be monitored. However, we shouldn't suppress them either because they are essential to our optimum decision making or, in some situations, like critical or emergency cases, cannot be replaced by analytical thinking. Thus, our real option is to strengthen our intuitions so that they become more accurate and provide us with better insights. Although intuitions may not always be reliable, they at least guide us in the right direction.

SHOULD WE TAKE GUT FEELINGS SERIOUSLY?

You had better take gut feelings seriously, as those feelings are borne out of your experience. Just because they are not conscious, we should not dismiss them. There are some limitations of conscious processes. You can only be conscious of one thing at a time. That's why consciousness is a bottleneck. Think about the differences between foveal vision and peripheral vision. If you didn't have peripheral vision, you would have great difficulty in walking, driving and orienting. Peripheral vision can be equated to subconscious thinking. In many situations, conscious analysis of choices does not work. Either there is not enough information, or there is too much information. If there is enough information, it may not be in the right form, or there isn't time to sort through it all. If we couldn't fall back on intuition, we would get stuck much of the time. Intuition lets us stay on cognitive autopilot so that we can focus on other important things at that moment. Intuition enables us to respond to the cues we're barely aware of. Intuition lets us size up situations in just a few seconds, and also provides early warnings of dangers.

There is some evidence that, when people ignore intuition, the quality of their decisions goes down. Surgery examinees experience this while solving multiple-choice questions in an examination. One of the explanations for this phenomenon is that some decisions are made subconsciously, before people even start to perform analysis, and the very act of articulating the factors can make decisions inappropriate. Some research has shown that people do worse at decision tasks when they are asked to perform analysis of the reason for their preferences, or to evaluate all the attributes of the choices.

Although intuition has its own limitations, it seems that we have made too much of them. Views such as 'intuition is basically untrustworthy' or 'avoid intuition at all costs' are going a bit too far. Going back to the analogy of the visual system, our eyes are not perfect. They have blind spots and sometimes require lenses to correct for distortion. Yet we don't reject the information we receive from our eyes. Similarly, just because intuition is fallible, that doesn't mean we can't make good use of it.

BLENDING ANALYSIS AND INTUITION

Neither analysis nor intuition alone is sufficient for every clinical decision that needs to be made. Therefore, we need to explore the connection between them, highlighting what can go wrong if we rely excessively on intuition and what can go wrong if we rely too much on analysis. The synthesis between intuition and analysis that seems most effective is when we put intuition in the driver's seat so that it directs our analysis of our circumstances. This way, intuition helps us recognise situations and helps us decide how to react, while analysis verifies our intuitions to make sure they aren't misleading us. Experts in this field recommend starting with intuition, not with analysis. If you begin by analysing a decision, you are inevitably going to suppress your intuition. You are better off starting by getting a sense of your intuitive preference – a gut check of your immediate preference, identifying your intuition before it gets clouded.

Pattern matching provides the initial understanding and recognition of how to react to a particular event, and the mental simulation (imagining how the reaction will play out) provides the deliberate thinking – the analysis – to help us decide if that course of action really would work. A good example of this process is, once again, our visual system. The fovea lets us see fine details. When we read, we focus the fovea on the letters. In contrast, peripheral vision is useful for providing the overall perspective that lets us keep ourselves well oriented in space. We need both the fovea and the periphery to carry on our lives. Of the two, the peripheral-vision system is more important. Our intuition functions like our peripheral vision, keeping us oriented and aware of our surroundings. Our analytical abilities, on the other hand, function like foveal vision and enable us to think precisely. We may believe that everything we think and decide comes from our analytical thinking, the conscious and deliberate arguments we construct in our heads, but that is because we are not aware of how our intuition directs our conscious thought processes.

Sometimes we need to rely more on intuition and other times we need to draw on analysis. When the situation keeps changing, when the time pressure is high, or when the aims are fuzzy, you cannot use analysis alone. You have to depend on your intuition. And when you have a lot of experience you can recognise what to do without having to weigh up all the options. In contrast, if you have to find the best option to solve a problem and not just a workable one, you may want to analyse the strengths and weaknesses of each alternative. If you have made a decision but are pressed to justify your choice, the most convincing way is to line up your options and explain why your selection was the wisest choice.

In chess, it is important to find the best move, not just a good one, so players continue to search for the best option. Yet it is also seen that, for the most part, they settle on the first option they had thought of, even after considering many others. It is likely that the first option that you think of while making a decision is the best. Although the results cannot be guaranteed, the observation is backed up by research evidence. Thus, it is important to note your initial impulse when faced with a difficult question. You should think about this option critically. You may discard it after a thought. But, if you ignore it, you would be missing out on some fast and free advice from your subconscious mind. And after thinking through your decision, if you really can't choose between different options, you should probably just go with the first impulse. A warning comes with this advice: do not mix up intuitions with desires. Sometimes, those first impulses are about what we want to have happen rather than what is likely to happen!

COGNITIVE AUTOPSY

Experience is a powerful teacher, but experience by itself is not the most efficient way to learn. The process can often be painful and time consuming. To learn as quickly as possible, we must be more deliberate, more disciplined and more thorough in our approach, in order to squeeze as much as possible from each experience. We can treat any experience as an opportunity to learn. There are a number of ways to get feedback about our decisions.

We often give feedback to ourselves. It is natural for us to mull over our decisions after the fact. We often beat ourselves up over bad decisions and congratulate ourselves for good ones. We often dwell on 'what if'. One of the most valuable things we can do is to take this natural tendency and refine and discipline it. Nevertheless, instead of passing judgement about whether it was a good decision or a bad decision, we should focus on understanding the decision process: why we decided what we did and how we made the decision. This type of feedback will give you a chance to revise and improve on your intuitions. When you do not have many chances to encounter challenging situations, you have to get the most out of the incidents you have. That means spending time afterwards to see what the incident has taught you. This applies both to real experiences and experiences from other or theoretical discussions and case examples in the books. Reflecting on our decisions is particularly useful when we have encountered some difficulty, including cases of failure. Failures grab and hold our attention, and they are loud signals that our mental models were not good enough. Failures hurt and that keeps us from forgetting them.

There are two types of feedback – the first is outcome feedback, which means that the decision makers are informed about the outcome of their decisions. In the case of surgical decisions, it means whether the action resulted in a positive outcome or not. The other kind of feedback is process feedback, which involves reflecting on how we made decisions and how we could have spotted patterns more quickly. Research has shown that we learn significantly better from process feedback and learn much less from outcome feedback. There is an important point to note here. Poor outcomes are different from poor decisions. The best decision possible given the knowledge available can still turn out unsatisfactorily. A poor decision is one for which we regret the process we used, in the following way: a person will consider a decision to be poor if the knowledge gained would lead to a different decision if a similar situation arose in future. Knowing simply that the outcome was unfavourable should not matter. Knowing what you failed to consider would matter.

In addition to feedback, expertise is affected by the opportunity to reflect on experiences. For example, chess masters do not spend all their time playing games against each other. The bulk of their time is spent studying the positions of previous games. During a tournament, a grandmaster will be working against the clock and will not be reflecting on the implications of the game, but afterwards there is time to go over the game record to look for opportunities that were missed, early signs that were not noticed or assessments and assumptions that were incorrect. In this way, an experience (even a single game) can be recycled and reused. In many field settings where there are limited opportunities to gain experience, developing the discipline of reviewing the decision-making process for each incident can be valuable.

We have a system already in place to learn from our experiences and to conduct post-mortems of our decisions: morbidity and mortality meetings. However, we find that the sessions typically get into debates about facts and details and ignore the practical or intuitive decision-making perspective. Instead of brainstorming sessions, they turn into blamestorming sessions. That is like giving people feedback on their driving by listing the cars they hit, without checking out their vision. Ideally, a good session would include a discussion of what was done. But it will also help people to learn about patterns – for instance, when was a problem first spotted, and were there earlier signs that were ignored? How were people interpreting the situation – were there different ideas about what was going on? What happened to make it clear? Could people have obtained more information earlier to reduce uncertainty? Did they wait too long, in the hope that uncertainty would diminish, and should they have acted more quickly to gain an advantage?

MANAGING CLINICAL UNCERTAINTY

Is clinical uncertainty inevitable? Clearly, the technology available in the future will dramatically increase the information available, yet we cannot be optimistic that increasing information will necessarily reduce uncertainty. It is more likely that the information age will change the challenges posed by uncertainty. Previously, information was missing because no one had collected it; in the future, information will be missing because no one can find it! Moreover, improved data collection will likely transform into faster decision cycles. By way of analogy, when radar was introduced into commercial shipping, it was with the intent of improving safety, so that ships could avoid collisions when visibility was poor. The actual impact was that ships increased their speed, and accident rates stayed constant. On the decision front, we expect to find the same thing. Planning cycles will be expedited and plans will be made with the same level of uncertainty as there was before. Moreover, people will expect faster decisions, without the time allowed in the past for thoughtful reflection.

Because uncertainty is inevitable, decisions can never be perfect. Often, we believe that we can improve the decision by collecting more information, but in the process we lose opportunities. Even if you gather information, key pieces may be missing, unreliable, ambiguous, inconsistent, or too complex to interpret, and as a result a decision maker will be reluctant to act. Because it is impossible to achieve 100% certainty, decision makers must be able to proceed without having a full under-standing of events. Skilled decision makers appear to know when to wait and when to act. Most importantly, they accept the need to act despite uncertainty.

In 1996, the world chess champion, Garry Kasparov, defeated the IBM chess computer Deep Blue in a six-game match. Observers noted that Deep Blue never adjusted its playing style. It always searched for the best move, even in positions where it knew it was behind. A human would have used intuitive thinking with a strategy that was speculative, rather than marching off to defeat. One of the IBM team members explained that the computer did not have a sense of 'creative desperation' – the sense that drives chess players to search for intuitive decisions, no mat-ter how risky.

Similar comment can be made about some surgeons while making decisions in stressful situations. They stick to a protocol rather than using intuitive decisions, although following the protocol may not be the best thing for the patient in that situation. If you do not make an effort to develop intuitive decision-making skill, you will not be able to make a decision in critical situations where it is most useful. Not being able to make an appropriate decision at a critical juncture may mean the outcome is not satisfactory, which may dent your confidence about making a decision. When a similar situation arises in future, you will feel very stressed while facing the situation; this will further affect your capacity to make good decisions. To avoid this downward spiral, it is helpful to build intuitive decision-making skill that you can rely on in difficult situations.

SUMMARY

One of the most important effects of acute stress is on decision-making capacity. Decision making lies at the heart of our surgeons' profes-sional lives. Decisions made by intelligent, responsible professionals during stressful situations can mean things go wrong. Unless we make conscious efforts to sharpen our intuitive skills, we may not be able to perform effectively and efficiently in stressful situations. Guidelines and protocols have a certain place in management. But they quickly fall apart when you need to think outside the box, and when symptoms are vague or multiple and the investigations are inconclusive. Neither analysis nor intuition alone is sufficient for every clinical decision that needs to be made. Therefore, we need to explore the connection between them, highlighting what can go wrong if we rely excessively on intuition and what can go wrong if we rely too much on analysis. In addition to feedback, expertise is affected by the opportunity to reflect on experiences.

REFERENCES

1 Groopman J. *How Doctors Think*. New York: Houghton Mifflin Company; 2007. p. 156.

2 Gawande A. *Complications: a surgeon's notes on an imperfect science*. New York: Henry Holt & Company; 2002.

3 Patkin M., Isabell L. Ergonomics, engineering and surgery of endo-surgical dissection. *J R Coll Surg Edinb*. 1995; 40: 120–32.

4 Klein G. *Sources of Power: how people make decisions*. Cambridge, MA: MIT Press; 1999. p. 35.

5 Benner P., Tanner C. How expert nurses use intuition. *Am J Nursing*. 1987; 87: 23–31.

6 Abernathy C.M., Hamm R.M. *Surgical Intuition: what it is and how to get it*. Philadelphia: Hanley & Belfus; 1994. pp. 102–42.

7 Wilson T.D., Schooler J.W. Thinking too much: introspection can reduce the quality of preferences and decisions. *J Pers Soc Psychol*. 1991; 60: 181–92.

8 Berlinger N.T. Vital signs: the breath of life. *Discover*. 1996; 17(3): 102–4.

CHAPTER 11

Epilogue

In 2009, US Airways flight 1549 took off from New York with 155 people on board. Immediately after take-off, it struck a large flock of Canada geese and both engines shut down. It is not unusual for planes to hit birds, but a dual bird strike is rare. Jet engines are designed to cope with most birds by liquefying them. However, because Canada geese are large, the engines shut down. Once the captain realised that both engines had failed, he took control of the plane and made an instinctive decision to carry out a crash landing on the Hudson River. All the passengers survived. After successfully landing the damaged Airbus on the Hudson River and saving the lives of all passengers, Captain Sullenberger was praised for his poise and calm demeanour during the crisis. When asked how he handled the situation so calmly, he responded, 'When I realised the crisis, I immediately took control and made a series of decisions. I thought that for the last forty-two years, I had been making small, regular deposits in the bank of "experience" by analysing and planning stressful situations, and on that day the balance was sufficient for me to make a large withdrawal.'

Have you ever thought about how to handle stress during critical incidents in the operating room? After reading thus far, if you haven't, you would be wise to do so. Of all the things that affect surgeons' performance, the inability to manage stress tops the list. Stress is a formidable issue for surgeons: it affects your professional life every day, often in a manner that you are not aware of, and after a certain stage it is detrimental to you. Inability to manage stress affects what we value most: technical skills, judgement, decision making and teamwork. It compromises your own integrity. Some surgeons say that they don't feel stressed. One of the reasons they do not feel stressed may be due to avoidance of stressful procedures rather than dealing with them. A few surgeons knowingly or unknowingly avoid performing operations that carry risk but offer better results for the patients. To avoid the stress, they may subject patients to sub-optimum treatment and compromise professional integrity.

You may have come across surgeons who are known to show grace under stressful situations and rise to the occasion. These are the experts we feel have nerves of steel and are immune to stress. They resemble elite athletes who perform with exceptional ability in the face of extreme pressure and rise above the anxieties and doubts that so often paralyse lesser performers. They retain the sureness of touch and subtlety of mind. No one appreciates this attitude better than trainees or residents who idolise these surgeons and consider them to be stress proof. The impression is that these surgeons perform – and excel – not in spite of stress, but *because* of it. As they say, 'pressure makes diamonds'.

To manage stress in this manner, what one needs to do is to leverage the natural stress management techniques each of us have to counteract the negative effects caused by pressure. When it comes to managing stress, many surgeons fail to use these techniques and handicap themselves. Insights regarding stress management have specific implications for every surgeon because individuals react to stress in predictable ways.

SWISS CHEESE MODEL OF ACCIDENTS

The Swiss cheese model (Figure 11.1) suggested by James Reason is useful to understand how untoward incidents happen during stressful situations while operating, even though we aim to reduce the incidences by taking different measures. He equated each defence system with a slice of cheese, a Swiss cheese to be specific. As you know, Swiss cheese has holes in it. James Reason likened the holes to the weaknesses of an individual or of defence systems. In a complex system like the operating room, we create barriers and place them in such a way that holes in each slice are covered by another slice so that the risk is not able to pass through the slices to cause damage by hitting the target. Thus the weakness in one individual is protected by another defence system.

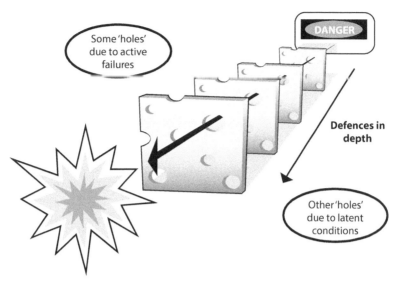

Figure 11.1 The Swiss cheese model. Source: Reproduced with permission from Flin R., Youngson G.G., Yule S. *Enhancing Surgical Performance: a primer in non-technical skills*. Boca Raton, FL: CRC Press; 2015.

For this reason, different individuals check and cross-check important documentation about a patient before taking them for the operation. It works most of the time. But these barriers are breached and a problem arises when the holes between the slices get aligned and risk factors pass through them. As Figure 11.1 shows, when the holes are not aligned, the danger is prevented by the slices.

James Reason described two types of event that cause defensive barriers to fail: active failures and latent conditions. In the first case, active failures, someone actively commits an act or error. In the case of latent conditions, there is an existing problem in the system that remains hidden until exposed by someone's actions. It can be said that latent conditions are like the hole in the slice getting wider and active failure is like someone moving the slice for the alignment to occur.

Stress is unique in the sense that it may act in both ways: as a latent condition as well as an active failure. Stress can cause the cheese to melt and widen a hole, as well as make you lose your grip on the slice and so allow it to be displaced and alignment to occur. If you look at the dynamics in the operating suite, as an operating surgeon, you are the last slice or barrier. You have a capacity to keep the hole (that is, stress), as narrow as you can and also hold it firmly to prevent the alignment from happening.

TEAM PERFORMANCE UNDER STRESS

It is not just individual surgeons whose performance is affected by stress; the performance of a whole team is affected. There is a view that teams perform well when stakes are highest. Nonetheless, like individuals, teams have a threshold for optimum performance. They don't necessarily perform well under stress. It is seen that when under pressure, teams get caught up with the trepidations of failure. The group thinking worsens and instead of choosing apt and unique solutions to the situation, the teams regress to sub-optimal approaches and run-of-the-mill solutions. They resort to ticking the boxes and perform at a minimum required level rather than stretching for additional effort.

In a stressful situation, the teams become over-dependent on a member who is at the highest level of hierarchy. This happens at the expense of another member who may be more suitable to handle the crisis but is not at the highest level. In the case of surgical teams, the operating surgeon stands at the highest level. Thus in a critical situation, whether the surgeon has appropriate information about the situation or not, the responsibility gets thrown his way. In a well-known case of an elective nasal surgery, an anaesthetist tried to intubate a patient but failed to insert the tube even after repeated attempts. Everybody in the operating room became stressed and focused attention to explore different ways to intubate the patient. They became so engrossed in trying to intubate that they were not able to pick up the seriously low hypoxic status. If they had noticed the hypoxia in time, alternative measures such as a tracheostomy could have taken place. Unfortunately, the patient died due to cerebral hypoxia.[1] During the debriefing of this case it became apparent that although it was an anaesthetic issue and while the nursing staff were ready with the tracheostomy set, the decision making was left only to the surgeon, who due to tunnel vision and other factors did not think of performing the tracheostomy and no other person took the decision.

As the critical issue around the stressful situation worsens, so does the group thinking. The group thinking becomes so narrowly focused that the consensus decision may sometimes overlook vital information. Specialised expertise gets ignored. In the case of the operating theatre, it may be someone like an anaesthetist, a scrub nurse or an assisting surgeon who has the expertise. In these situations, group thinking may mean taking mediocre and soft options rather than bold unconventional measures.

What can you do?

If there is a one essential strategy for performing according to your capability in a stressful moment, it is to minimise the harmful effects of stress on you. Since it is impossible to function as a surgeon without stress, the key is to negotiate your reactions, gain insight into how stress affects you and then plan techniques to manage it. You cannot change how much stress you are going to face, but you can change how to deal with the stress by providing yourself with the techniques to become more effective under pressure. I have observed surgeons who under stressful situations are able to perform well. They still experienced stress, and they still were negatively affected by stress, but just like successful performers in other domains, they were able to manage it more effectively. Surgeons who falter less under stress than others have a different road map for handling stress than those who try to do so unsuccessfully. They use specific strategies to perform to the best of their capability. These strategies develop from natural faculties. These faculties are thoughts, physiological responses, perceptual sensations and bodily actions. Managing and improvising these faculties determine how you handle stress. An important point to note, the skill of improvising the (stress-related) faculties is unrelated to your level of expertise.

Surgeons who handle stress better are appropriately sensitive to their physiological arousal changes that help them regulate their bodily mechanisms. They do this sometimes consciously but most of the times unconsciously. For example, breathing slower at the time of crisis enables them to process information effectively and prevent impulsive decisions. Regulating physiological arousal is important if one wants to manage emotions such as anxiety and impulsiveness. Learning to use natural faculties each of us has can help you to manage the demands that stress puts on you.

Unlike other stress-prone disciplines, surgeons are not offered systematic guidance for effectively dealing with stress. Consequently, inexperienced surgeons are not explicitly taught how to manage intraoperative stressors when they occur. They learn to cope only through observing others managing similar scenarios or from making their own mistakes; that is, by trial and error. As with the acquisition of other skills, such unsystematic learning is not appropriate anymore for various reasons. First, without effective feedback and explanation of why the other surgeon acted in a certain manner, it is hard for you to understand what is going on. Second, the time available for learning by experience is diminishing. The first time that surgeons encounter a particular stressful situation may be when they are responsible for dealing with it; hardly a situation appropriate either as a learning environment or in providing safe patient care. To address the deficiency, here are a few common and effective strategies that I was able to obtain from surgeons experienced in handling stressful situations in the operating room.

- **Look at stressful moments as a challenge or opportunity:** People differ in their approach of looking at a stressful situation. Some look at it as a threatening situation while others see it as a challenge. Some people embrace these moments while others dread them. Perceiving stressful situations as a threat undermines self-confidence and elicits fear of failure, impairs working memory and attention and makes you vulnerable to impulsive behaviour. On the other hand, individuals who perceive the situation not as a threat but as a challenge are far more likely to perform to their level of ability, increasing their chances of success. When they see the stressful situation as a challenge, they are stimulated to give the attention and energy needed to make the best efforts. The physiological arousal is experienced as exciting rather than uncomfortable and unsettling. When you see surgeons who tackle a difficult complication while performing a critical surgery, you can assume that they are not thriving on a stressful situation as you thought. Rather, they are thriving on a challenging situation. The things that they say to themselves are along the lines of, 'I want to see how good I can be in this situation.'

- **A critical situation is one of many opportunities:** They neither look at the critical situation as a 'do or die' episode nor look at it as if the world will end if they do not handle it satisfactorily. They assure themselves of getting more than one chance to make it right. This self-assurance reduces their stress.

- **Shrinking the importance of the stressful moment:** It is a known experience that the more important we evaluate an event to be, the more stressful we find it. The stress distorts our perception, and these distorted perceptions affect judgement and decision making. One can reduce the stress of the moment by minimising its significance.

Someone may comment that it is unrealistic to say that something is not really important when you know it really is. Understanding that is it is equally unrealistic to exaggerate the significance refutes this comment. It is a common tendency to exaggerate when you are in a stressful situation. When you minimise the situation you negate the effect of distortion and gain realistic perspective by counteracting the exaggeration.

- **Maintaining focus on the ultimate goal:** Experts stay clear on what they are trying to achieve. For them the task is part of the ultimate goal to use skill and knowledge in the best possible way to help the patient in front of them. Increasing this awareness of the ultimate goal before and during stressful moments helps to destress the situation. First, it prevents disturbing thoughts created by self-consciousness or outer distractions. Second, keeping an eye on the mission keeps you on track because it guides you to do things you need to do to achieve the performance you are aiming for. One needs to be aware that focusing on the goal is different from focusing on the outcome or positive results. If you focus on outcome you will end up with the thoughts of negative consequences if you do not achieve the positive result. Thinking about not achieving what you desire will make you more anxious and worsen the stress. On the other hand, focusing on the ultimate goal creates a mindset that will find the best way to accomplish the task.

- **Know the difference between positive stress and negative stress:** Why do some people feel that stress is helpful for performance while others think it is unhelpful? It is understandable why we have this question. The term stress itself gives a negative connotation so how can one consider it to be positive? Stress, in the broadest sense, is a reaction to the demands being made on an individual. This definition does not automatically equate to a negative state. When the demands of the situation exceed the individual's capacity to handle them appropriately, the stress is negative.

The ability to achieve the optimum state between positive and negative stress is an attribute that we observe in experts. The physiological changes that we experience, increased heart rate or rapid breathing, are similar in both positive as well as negative stressful situations. But we can differentiate between them according to the consequences or seriousness of the outcome. In other words, negative stressful situations may have the same physiological effects but they are different from positive stressful situations, as the outcome of your actions is critical or a matter of life and death. These are the situations where you feel that something at stake is dependent on your performance. While positive stressful moments are important, the outcome is not perceived as critical. In short, the fight and flight response does not need to be activated when stress is positive.

There is a specific evolutionary function for positive stress and negative stress. Since ancient times, humans have had demands placed on us by the environment. Meeting those demands, such as seeking food and shelter or looking after offspring, required effort and time, so a stress response evolved that would set off a chemical reaction to get those things done. It prepares the body to meet the demands, thus positive stress helped us to maintain survival. Negative stress developed differently. It evolved as a 'selection mechanism' – to decide who would advance in life and who would not. To escape a predator chasing you is more than a positively stressful situation; either you find a way to escape or to fight the predator, or you potentially will die. In case of negative stress, something critical is on the line. For primitive humans, their life was on the line – failure to escape would result in death. 'I have to succeed or else' was a right judgement of the situation, but today it is best described as a negative stressful response that will derail you in a critical situation. When you become aware of these differences, it will allow you to react more proportionally to the kind of situation you are facing. Thus every action that you take in the operating room should not necessarily carry life-or-death consequences. Yes, there are situations that may have dire consequences but not in every case. Those surgeons who have this proportionality appear to be confident yet humble, positive yet realistic.

In the inverted U graph (Figure 11.2), the vertical axis represents level of performance, while the horizontal axis represents the level of stress. There is a peak in the middle. To the left side of the peak is positive stress and to the right side is negative stress. The left-hand side of the graph shows the situation where people are under-challenged, are not experiencing any stress. Here they are not geared up to do their best and hence performance is 'sloppy'. With some stress, which is positive at this stage, performance starts improving until it reaches a peak. The right-hand side of the graph shows where we start falling apart under stress (i.e. negative stress). Due to the various factors in the operating room, you may be already sitting at the top when you start the procedure, so when you are faced with the added stress, your performance

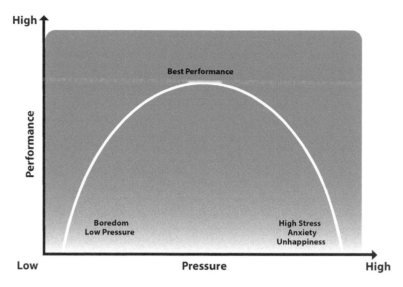

Figure 11.2 The inverted U model explains the variance between positive and negative stress.

deteriorates. Think of a computer analogy: if a computer is running several programs at once, each of the programs runs slower and is prone to crash. In the middle of the graph you perform at peak effectiveness. You are sufficiently motivated to work hard, but not so overloaded as to start struggling. This is where a surgeon enters in a state of 'flow' – the enjoyable and highly productive state in which you do your best work.

Have you ever been so involved in performing a procedure that you lost track of time? Everything around you – from ringing of phones to the noisy conversation among the staff – seemed to fade away? Your attention was focused entirely on what you were doing and you were engrossed in the procedure? You felt energised about what you were doing? If you have experienced this feeling, you have experienced an optimum stress-free performance – 'flow'. In a flow you are so focused on a task that everything else falls away ... action and awareness merge ... time flies ... the self vanishes ... performance goes through the roof. Flow is a state we reach when our perceived skills match the perceived challenge. When we are in a state of flow, the performance fills us with joy and we lose our sense of self as we concentrate fully on the task. This is the state we're in when we're at our most productive.

If the task isn't challenging, we are likely to feel indifferent towards it. But facing challenging tasks without the required skills could cause stress. To find a balance and to perform at our best, we need a challenge that is significant and interesting and we need well-developed skills, so that we are confident that we can meet the challenge. This moves us to a position where we experience flow. This is the state that I have observed in expert surgeons performing most of the time. This should be an aim of every surgeon before entering the operating room. As mentioned above, there must be a good balance between your perceived skill and the perceived challenge of the task. If one of these weighs more heavily than the other, flow probably won't occur. Remember that simply increasing the amount of challenge doesn't guarantee flow. You experience flow only when you perceive the right opportunities. It happens because you're in the right mindset, not because you have 'perfect conditions'.

We call this experience flow because that is the sensation conferred. In flow, every action and every decision leads effortlessly, fluidly and seamlessly to the next. It's being swept along by the river of ultimate performance. It transforms a weakling into a muscleman, a sketcher into an artist, an ordinary performer into someone extraordinary. Everything you do, you do better in flow, from tissue handling to decision making to maintaining situation awareness. You could say that flow is the doorway to the 'best' room most of us seek.

Flow is a transformation available to anyone, anywhere, provided certain conditions are met. Cognitive scientists now believe flow sits at the heart of almost every optimum performance. Yet there is a rub. Flow might be the most desirable state; it's also the most elusive. We know that our performance needs to be at peak, but we still don't know the exact optimal conditions for flow for an individual surgeon for a specific procedure. Hopefully, the understanding you have received after reading this book will create an insight to achieve the 'flow'. Flow is the hallmark of high performance, but in situations where the slightest error could be fatal, perfection is the only choice – and flow is the only guarantee of perfection.

To achieve flow in a consistent manner you need to manage stress in a consistent manner. As it has been done, we took the first step by becoming aware and acknowledge the issue of stress among surgeons, then obtained the facts about stress affecting surgical performance. In the later part we saw the specific factors that precipitates stress. In addition to the ergonomic measures that one should consider to reduce stress, we saw specific strategies to improve operative skills and decision-making skills. As mentioned at the start, by assimilating this information and implementing the suggestions, you will be using the cutting-edge results from what cognitive science has to offer. When you apply these strategies, in stressful situations, you will experience less distorted and distracted thinking, less indecision and more creativity. I believe that when you walk into an operating room to perform a very complex procedure, you will see that as more of a challenge than a crisis, and after the procedure you will walk away feeling confident that you performed in a way closer to what you are capable of, not less. Helping you to experience the 'flow' while operating has been the purpose behind writing this book and I hope that you will be able to accomplish it.

REFERENCE

1 Bromily M. Have you ever made a mistake? *RCOA Bulletin*. 2008; 48: 2242–5.

Index